Autonomy in Nursing

Mary O'Neil Mundinger, R.N., M.A.

Graduate Division of Nursing
Family Nurse Practitioner Program

Pace University
Briarcliff Manor, New York

Aspen Systems Corporation
Germantown, Maryland
London, England
1980

Library of Congress Cataloging in Publication Data

Mundinger, Mary O'Neil.
Autonomy in nursing.

Includes bibliographies and index.

1. Nursing—Philosophy.   2. Nursing—Practice.
3. Autonomy.   4. Nurse practitioners. I.   Title.
RT85.5.M86   610.73'01   79-25630
ISBN: 0-89443-171-4

Library of Congress Catalog Card Number: 79-25630
ISBN: 0-89443-171-4

Printed in the United States of America

1 2 3 4 5

To Paul, with love

Table of Contents

Foreword

Regardless of the specific phraseology individuals may use, the concept of autonomy is one of the primary concerns of professional nurses. It is, indeed, the hallmark of professionalism and is a clear delineation of *professional* nursing practice that has major implications for all nurses.

Why the problem? Aren't nurses generally accepted as professionals? Doesn't everyone know what nurses do? The answer to both questions tends to be: just to a certain extent. Certainly state licensure identifies them legally as professional nurses, but for historical and economic reasons they have been identified so closely with medicine and hospitals that many people still think that the most important aspect of nursing is carrying out doctors' orders.

Hospital employed nurses are the largest group of working nurses and therefore the most visible, and the care they give is seen as illness-oriented and physician-directed. Even the dramatic actions of coronary care nurses are viewed by many as substitutes for the physician's decision rather than the autonomous decisions that they actually are. Moreover, in the closely structured, bureaucratic, institutional environment, with patients attended by teams rather than individuals, accountability always seems to be at least one person away.

Only when the nurse practitioner emerged and was publicized to a great extent as a rather independent practitioner in areas with minimal available health care was there some recognition that this person really drew from a body of professional knowledge and then used the necessary judgment to make autonomous decisions about the care of patients. Once more, however, the picture was fogged by the medical focus of some of the care. Some nurses approved it; some did not; but the question of whether any aspect was autonomous *nursing* practice was frequently raised.

Perhaps the problem is intensified because so many nurses simply cannot identify the uniqueness of nursing, and those who can have a tendency to shroud it in theoretical terms. In this book, the author presents in a straightforward, down-to-earth way, her concept of independent nursing practice and identifies clearly its elements. The settings are varied; independent practice has no situational limits. But the components of individual decision making are the same.

This is a thought-provoking and challenging book. The reader will be referring back to certain sections time and time again to reconsider and rethink old notions about what professional practice is. No matter who holds these notions—practicing nurses or students, physicians, or the public —and no matter whether they are reinforced, enlarged, or discarded, one result is bound to occur: readers will develop an appreciation of the tremendous impact professional nursing has on health care when autonomous practice is the mode, not the exception.

Lucie S. Kelly, R.N., Ph.D., F.A.A.N.
Professor of Nursing
(in Public Health)
Director of Nursing Programs
School of Public Health and
School of Nursing
Columbia University

Acknowledgments

Two groups of people have made this volume possible: professional nursing colleagues who gave creative support and leadership to first the vision and then the reality of autonomous practice and my family, who have not only encouraged me in my work but also willingly accepted the sacrifices that it entailed.

Grace Jauron refined many of the beginning concepts and was responsible for important insights regarding the nature of autonomous practice. Sue Helstein and Virginia Baker worked closely with us to transform some of these ideas into a primary nursing system. My later interests in family nurse practitioner work and community nursing grew out of our initial and exciting collaboration. Special thanks go to Sylvia Carlson, who early and dynamically showed us all the beginnings of primary nursing and autonomous practice. The nurses with whom we all worked deserve praise and thanks for their commitment in adopting the new models of practice and thereby enriching the health care for their clients.

During the writing of this book, my four teen-aged children moved into high school or college and helped with many of my family responsibilities so that I could continue. My husband provided the suggestions, support, and encouragement that made the project a happy and rewarding one. My loving thanks go to each of them.

Introduction

This is a book about professional nursing and how it happens in a variety of settings. Although focused on individual nurses and the mastery of their profession, the information here can be valuable to administrators and educators in nursing as well. The development of professional accountable and autonomous practice is more assured when the leadership as well as the practitioners have full and knowledgeable commitment to the same ideal.

The criteria for development as a professional are discussed, and one view of autonomy is presented. The nursing process as the methodical way to identify, plan, and give and evaluate effective nursing care is demonstrated in a number of case studies. Using this design, a nurse can put professional care into effect for clients, even without administrative recognition or support. The roles of primary nurse, nurse practitioner, and community nurse are presented as examples of professional practice. Examples of actual client-nurse interactions are given, with identification of the nursing diagnoses and therapy. The traditional medical extension of the nurse practitioner is challenged, with a focus instead on the complex management of chronic illness, which might be more appropriate and effective when provided by nurse practitioners than by physicians. The historical public health nurse role is seen as self-limiting and in need of renewal, with extension toward primary care, independent problem resolution, and a broader community clientele. Primary nursing, the third model, is the nursing framework that must be used to meet the requirements of hospitalized patients. With shorter hospital stays and stricter admission criteria, a greater percentage of patients are acutely ill and in need of comprehensive and professionally expert care every hour of their hospital stay.

Nursing is moving quickly, creatively, and in exciting ways toward new requirements for professional practice. Nursing's maturity will be marked by the acceptance of the professional service of nursing as not only separate and distinct, but also as a necessary component of health care. Without identity there can be no survival and no collaboration. Not only is this philosophically true, but it is also a critical issue today.

Nursing is experiencing dissension and decay within its own ranks, which is compromising its distinction as a profession. Without consensus within nursing about its competencies and purpose, there can be no identity. As this argument goes on unresolved, health care decisions and priorities are being made nationally that should include a strong and unified component of professional nursing. Many who want to include nursing as a major part of health care delivery and direction are waiting for nursing to state its skill, objectives, accountability, and turf. This book is designed to assist in that effort. Not only must the autonomous aspects of nursing service (the professional component) be identified, but they must also be expanded, with a changing focus from illness care to health care. This can happen in one of two ways: one, by the medical profession assuming direction for health-promotive and illness-preventive care and bringing nursing along as an assistive function; and, two, by nursing asserting its legitimate leadership and autonomy in those areas, and collaborating with the medical profession in a true team effort. It seems to me that the latter will be more productive and complete, and certainly more satisfying for both the people served and for the nurses. Physicians, in time, may recognize the benefits that are clearly theirs, too, in such a system.

Chapter 1

Autonomy: The Significance for Client and Nurse

Those of us who are pioneers in the field of developing and establishing autonomous nursing practice constantly are defending our work to those who believe we should be involved instead in a shared team effort to define and treat health problems, on the ground that this is in the client's best interest. Autonomy is a concept about independence, identity, and authority. It is a necessary attribute of professional practice. Without autonomy nursing service can be limited according to the perspective and objectives of the one directing nursing. Only a nurse knows when nursing is needed, and without autonomy, the existence of that service is in jeopardy. Autonomy is not synonomous with isolation, and it is not situational: autonomous practice can be interdependent (two or more dependent practices interweaving for enhancement of each) and it can happen regardless of the setting. Autonomous nursing care is a concept about theory-based practice and accountable, authoritative decision making.

Autonomous practice happens whenever a nurse makes an independent judgment about the presence of a health problem and then provides the resolution through nursing care. It can happen in any setting regardless of the presence or absence of a medical crisis or condition, and it can include collaborative plans and actions with other professionals and health care workers. Autonomy means identity (form, not shadow), independence (ability to stand alone), and authority (theory and rationale for practice acknowledged by others). Autonomy operationally is power.

This book is designed to share with professional nurses the reasons and methods for establishing autonomy in nursing practice in a variety of settings. It also is an effort to demonstrate, with examples, how this comprehensive practice of professional nursing functions. By identifying what nurses are most competent in providing, the service clients need and receive can be established. This is necessary for the survival of professional

1

nursing. Only when we isolate the components and outcomes of such services can we assure our clients that they will not be lost within the confines and priorities of other health care practices. Then we can join in a shared effort for health care.

An effective team effort for health care will occur only when all team members identify their areas of expertise and accept accountability for providing those services. Those separate identities then can form a strong coalition for health: "On a real team everyone functions in a primary role."[1] If, instead, nursing were to answer the call for teamwork before identifying and demonstrating its special mission, there would be a real danger that professional nursing services would not be available in the team package. For if nurses cannot name those services, how can we expect the health team to provide them? And if nurses cannot say what those services are, we cannot say when they are absent. Without this identity, we cannot expect to function as team leaders—a role it will be appropriate for them to assume at times. Therefore, to ensure the survival of nursing services for clients, those services must be identified. This is the primary reason for the effort to develop autonomous nursing service.

THE RIVALRY FOR AREAS OF PRACTICE

Today many new health care workers are laying claim to practice areas that were nursing's in the past. Some not-so-new health care workers are expanding their territories onto nursing turf as well. This is happening at a time when we in nursing are just beginning to emerge as consciously committed professionals.

It is imperative for our clients that we work now to establish the field of therapy that is unique to nursing and to see that it is identified in the legal definitions of nursing practice everywhere. We need to work for legislation that will identify the specific nursing therapies so that we can provide them legally, have them recognized as our own privilege and responsibility, and be reimbursed independently for them—the fee for service. And we need to develop modes of practice so we can indeed provide those services to our clients.

A professional generally is thought to be one educated to provide essential services to people. There is a theory and a practice element for all professions. Each has a unique area of theory-practice as well as shared areas. For instance, medicine, law, clergy, and education all have special and different curricula in their educational systems. Each also has a practice to offer and an internship for learning to put the theory to work. Certainly there are other occupations that combine knowledge/practice into a specialized service, such as plumbers, watch repairers, and engineers, but the professions differ in that they work with people. Each possesses a unique therapy, identifiably different from any of the other professions. Nursing always has had the first component identified—providing essential services to people—but has not identified what makes its practice different and unique. There are four major reasons for this:

1. Nurses have been allied very closely with medicine, and it is difficult for our outline to be seen in a shadow that looms so large.
2. Nurses usually are employees and not available for initial and direct contact with clients or for outlining their own priorities of care once contact is made.
3. Nursing's educational system often has been closer to an apprenticeship than to an internship—the functions are learned without the underlying theory.
4. The results of nurses' interventions often are more subtle, short term, and less visible and dramatic than some other professional services.[2]

Nurses have an enormous task resolving these four issues, as well as a host of other problems. One is that we sometimes fail to recruit persons who value accountability, risk taking, and leadership. There are, unfortunately, many in our ranks who find great satisfaction in nonprofessional practice. How can a few nurses develop and identify one kind of practice if the majority continue to practice in another way? How can clients tell the difference and choose between them? Another problem is money. Are enough health care dollars available in this country to pay for professional nursing? If not, what are the compromises? What will the trade-offs be?

THE BASIS FOR NURSING'S ROLE

Components of professional practice are those things nurses know more about and do better than anyone else. Autonomous practice has to do with competence in why and when as well as how certain activities are carried out. We have been doing many things for our clients, and doing them well. What often has been missing is the initiation of those activities because we know their purpose and the clear accountability for what the outcome should be. One example is the positioning of patients. In a hospital postoperative setting, positioning often is written into physician's orders to nurses or in hospital routines: "Turn every 2 hours" or "elevate legs 30°." It isn't quite that simple, however. In actuality, nurses are doing far more. They are thinking about both the curative effect of such therapies (reducing edema, clearing secretions, etc.) and the preventive aspects (prevention of stasis, emboli, edema, pneumonia, decubiti). They know when to implement such therapies and when to modify or discontinue them. For instance, hemorrhage, pain, blood pressure or other condition changes would prompt nurses to reassess the situation. They know, too, how successful implementation and modification should result (improved circulation, decreased edema, improved respirations, absense of pain, etc.). And lastly, they know how to do the positioning more skillfully than anyone else.

Knowing why, when, and how to position clients and doing it skillfully makes the function an autonomous therapy. But, if physicians order it, how can it be autonomous? If physicians order an action nurses would not do in the absence of those orders, if they do not know why or when to do so, it probably is a dependent rather than autonomous function. But if the nurse has the knowledge and the skill to initiate and carry out the actions and answer for the results, then it is autonomous.

Many activities that historically were medical therapies have become nursing's. Every profession grows in the range of services as new needs and new technologies become known. Legal services for collective bargaining, educational services for dyslexia, and surgical techniques for joint replacements all are examples of expanding services in the professions. Because nursing has been seen for so long as an arm of medicine, most of its expanded services have been in the realm of medicine—blood pressures, venipunctures, cardiac defibrillation, and physical assessment, for instance. Nursing has not been expanding its own practice because it has not articulated what that practice is.

Perhaps in the future, as medical services expand, the delegation of lesser medical technologies will go instead to physician's assistants and free nurses to develop and expand nursing practice, with our own overflow going to our own aides or, better yet, to our clients. For an example, another look at positioning patients is appropriate. A nurse working in that hypothetical surgical unit has decided on the basis of his or her knowledge and skill that a certain client is an appropriate candidate for a positioning regimen. The nurse states the rationale, regime, and expected results, and proceeds. A not-so-hypothetical surgeon storms in and tells the nurse in no uncertain terms that if positioning is needed the surgeon will order it. The surgeon has no reasons to rebut the nurse's plan, it is just that, after all, it is the surgeon's client. Well, is it the surgeon's client for nursing care as well as for the medical care? Most physicians still think so. Some hospital administrators and nursing directors, however, are becoming aware that there should be a division of authority, with the physicians holding only a part of that power, although a major one.

Who is accountable for what in hospital care is being redefined in hospital policy and in the courts. The continuing problem is that nurses remain employees in the same institutions where physicians have very different kinds of relationships with clients. Perhaps clients need a system whereby they contract for certain services with a professional nurse when entering the hospital. Clients and physicians need to know what those services are. An example of contracted service is given by M. Lucille Kinlein in her book *"Independent Nursing Practice With Clients."*[3] Other examples appear in chapter 4 on primary nursing.

If autonomous nursing service involves those activities that nurses are best prepared to initiate and do, then what are dependent therapies? And are not some of these shared?

Dependent nursing practice includes actions nurses take at the initiation of another's orders or delegation, and because the knowledge and outcome of such activities falls within the scope and competency of that other profession. Generally, the director of care is the physician. A physician cannot make an autonomous nursing function a dependent one simply by adding it to the medical orders, such as positioning. However, when an autonomous nursing activity is influenced by medical factors, the nursing function may then become shared or dependent. Most nurses, by dint of practice and because of limitations imposed by employers, are most competent and comfortable in the not-so-unique, or dependent, skills of nursing. It is not that they value the nonprofessional aspects of nursing more than the professional ones, but nursing care priorities usually are set by nonnurses who cannot be adept at knowing the difference and providing time and resources for both.

The technical components of nursing are those identified most easily by employers, physicians, and clients. One reason is that medical practice is recognized easily and is valued by these three groups, while the nonprofessional (or dependent) functions of nursing are the less skilled medical care activities delegated or ordered by physicians. A second reason is that the technical functions of nursing are more visible and predictable in outcome. For instance, giving an injection for pain is an easily recognizable and acceptable nursing function for pain relief, as opposed to positioning, back rub, and counseling for what may indeed be pain of psychological origin.

Generally, three factors—competence, value, and comfort—are allied closely to activities in which individuals also have the most knowledge and skill. Therefore, given a variety of tasks, people rarely will compromise the ones they value and in which they have competence and comfort.

Dependent nursing functions generally fit into this three-fold category. Nurses value what their clients value, which historically has been medical care and not health care. The dependent functions are those in which nurses experience the most comfort and competence because they are the skills taught most thoroughly and practiced most often.

There also are times when the dependent care we give is directed by health professionals other than a physician. Again, think back to positioning. A client is postoperative for a fractured hip and has been referred by the surgeon to physiotherapy for a series of advanced weight-bearing exercises. The physiotherapist designs a regimen based on the type of fracture and repair and the client's stamina, body build, and degree of compliance. The regime should be carried out a number of times a day, sometimes by the nurse rather than the physiotherapist. In this instance, the dependent nursing activities were defined by a physiotherapist. Perhaps this same client will need convalescent care in another institution before returning home. The social worker, in determining placement, needs assistance from nursing in defining the client's self-care status. This, too, could be considered a dependent function. It also could be considered a shared function in that we nurses are best prepared to assess and define self-care abilities while the social worker is best prepared to use that information as one component in obtaining proper placement.

Under certain circumstances, the positioning therapies discussed also could be considered shared or dependent functions with medicine. The guiding criteria are whether or not the pathology (medical independent practice) impinges on the why, when, or how of a positioning routine. For instance, positioning a client with a fractured hip will be dependent or shared nursing therapy, whereas positioning purely for comfort or for preventative care is an autonomous nursing therapy.

Positioning is a therapy commonly practiced in the acute care setting, but there may be different priorities for care in the community. For example, skin care or counseling might be more common functions for discussion of community-based autonomous practice. Either the nurse or the client can identify skin care as a need. The nurse may identify actual skin problems such as dryness, cracking, decreasing circulation, open sores, rashes, abrasions, etc., or potential problems may be identified on the basis of activity (athlete's increased perspiration and friction), clothing (constricted or poorly fitted), medical condition (diabetes), or diet (decreased vitamin C or protein). The therapies used would be varied and related directly to the cause. Part of our work would be to assess the presence of any medical reason for a skin problem. Infection, medications, allergies, or existing disease (such as diabetes) all would indicate the need for sharing responsibility for the client with a physician. As with positioning, if there are no other health determinants of skin care, the nursing regimen becomes an autonomous one.

Healthy skin depends on a variety of factors ranging from adequate intake of protein and vitamins to absence of local irritants. Almost all skin care can be done by the client if the individual knows why and how. Since nursing is, to many, the potentiation of optimum self-care, skin care fits well into the autonomous nursing category.[4]

Essential therapies to assure cleanliness, circulation, and comfort can be carried out autonomously. When the cause of the skin problem involves shared therapy (the diabetic, the patient with peripheral vascular disease, or a collagen disease) the initial nursing therapies may be the same— cleaning open areas, using an antiseptic where indicated, exercising, positioning, wearing clothing to decrease constriction or dependency and to increase circulation, or applying heat, cold, analgesics, or other topical agents for comfort. The underlying cause of skin problems may not be pathological but may be due to such things as protein or other vitamin deficiencies, dry air, local allergens, or immobility. All of these causes, as well as the initial skin problem, can be treated autonomously by nurses.

Even when the underlying cause is pathological, much of nursing therapy still is autonomous. With the diabetic, foot care is more diligent, lesions are treated more aggressively, and the degree of diabetic control will influence skin integrity—but the nursing therapies do not change. They simply are instituted with different degrees of intensity and in collaboration with the medical plan, which is what makes skin care a shared therapy in the presence of pathology.

Massage is a useful and appropriate nursing measure for some skin problems. However, for the client with real or potential phlebitis or abnormal clotting times, massage would be contraindicated or done less aggressively—an example of dependent or medically directed (or limited) nursing practice.

THE ESTABLISHMENT OF AUTONOMOUS NURSING

The previous examples demonstrate autonomous nursing therapy in positioning or skin care. The reasons why identification of autonomous nursing therapies has been such a slow and confusing process were stated earlier:

1. nursing's close alliance with medicine
2. nurse's employee status and secondary access to clients
3. apprenticeship education
4. lack of definitive and permanent health outcomes

Although all four bear responsibility for nursing's hidden significance, only the second and third are likely to change. The close alliance with medicine has been detrimental in establishing a separate identity for nursing. Most nurses work in hospitals and most of the care is medically directed. Clients are admitted to hospitals by physicians for cure or relief of medical problems. The hospital serves as a technologically skilled and expensive area with 24-hour nursing and support care available. As clients' needs for these services decrease, they are discharged to a different setting. Because nursing problems rarely require expensive techniques and intensive continuous care, clients seldom will remain in the hospital for nursing therapy only. This produces a paradoxical situation in which nurses are most often found in the very setting where autonomous nursing therapy is a low priority for clients.

Client readiness for nursing therapy also is rarely synchronous with nursing availability. Even if we nurses were not completely occupied with medically directed care, clients often are not ready for autonomous nursing therapies in an acute care setting. Those hospitalized are acutely ill, and their energies and attention are focused on the crisis at hand. They may not be willing, able, or interested in addressing the preventive (self-) care that could assure nonrecurrence of that crisis, and they may have the same disinterest in rehabilitative and health-promoting activities until the current medical problem is resolved.

In most successful nursing care, the client is a participant. Doing with the client rather than doing to is far more descriptive of nursing than medicine. The clients' active involvement that goes on in effective nursing therapy requires their motivation, participation, and attention in order to work. This interaction usually cannot occur until the more pressing need—the medical problem—is solved. Most nursing care is given not only in a medical setting (a hospital) but also is seen as an adjunct to that medical care. Clients come in contact with nursing care through their medical treatment.

In most instances, nursing care is a reimbursable expense only when medical care is being delivered. All of this tends to reinforce the commonly held idea (and certainly that of most physicians) that nursing care is a totally medically dependent service. Any casual observer would think so, too. Not only is nursing seen most often in combination with medicine, but many of the functions look the same. Body inspections and treatment of symptoms are performed by both nurses and physicians. Even interviewing and the questions asked sound similar.

The idea that similar looking data collected by two dissimilar professions could be used in very different ways is alien to most persons. Surely the nurse with one stethoscope is doing the same thing as the physician. Or is it the same? Nurses must explain to clients and each other how their therapy, based on data from the stethoscope-to-abdomen maneuver, differs markedly from that resulting from the identical data gathering by a physician. Each may hear an absence of bowel sounds. For the physician, this may mean prostigmine injections and perhaps surgical intervention. For the nurse, a different therapeutic regime becomes apparent: positioning to relieve pressure from distension, ambulation to encourage gas mobilization, diet changes that could mean smaller meals or none at all (depending on bowel motility), and monitoring fluid and solid intake as well as urinary and stool output.

Similarly, when listening to breath sounds, both nurse and physician may hear exactly the same thing but prescribe and be accountable for different care. To the physician, rales in the bases of both lungs may suggest x-ray, antibiotics, and respiratory therapy. To the nurse, rales may suggest a different but certainly complementary plan: positioning and client teaching to assist deeper breathing, coughing and expectorating, smaller and more frequent meals so that diaphragmatic pressure upward from a full stomach will not hamper breathing further, increased fluid intake (unless other data were to suggest heart failure), and monitoring changes in vital signs, skin color and moisture, and respiration quality.

THERAPIES DIFFER

It becomes obvious from these examples that it is the different therapies that distinguish nursing from medicine, for there is much that is shared in the gathering of data.

In the nursing team, many therapies are shared by nonprofessional caregivers. Again, to the casual observer it would look as though a nurse and a nurse's aide were giving exactly the same care. Many nursing actions are identical to the close bodily care activities of everyday living. One would be hard put to distinguish on sight between the back rub given to a client by a professional nurse and the same activity by a nurse's aide or a practical nurse. How often is heard, "I do the same thing as the nurse," and that often is true. What is different is why an activity is carried out, what can be accomplished by doing it, and what further information can be learned through its actual performance. A back rub by any caring individual shows concern and promotes relaxation. The nurse's repertoire of therapy and information gathering is far richer. The professional back rub will yield data on circulation, respiratory quality, skin integrity, hair growth patterns, muscle tone and tenseness, and the presence of unusual lumps or lesions. It also will provide the opportunity for clients to voice their concerns — especially those they consider too unimportant for primary consultation time with the nurse.

Because clients easily identify physical nursing care such as back rubs, dressing changes, and bathing, these can be used successfully as a means of access to those who need a wider range of professional nursing care. Identification of professional nursing by clients still is so indistinct that they rarely seek it out.

A woman with terminal cancer returned home after lung surgery and asked me to do her dressing changes evenings when the public health nurse no longer was available. I did so for a number of weeks, and the ten minutes or so that the dressing change required gave me the opportunity to counsel her on her nutritional needs, listen to her brave and funny remarks about her self-care abilities, to answer her husband's whispered worried questions before I left for the night, and to offer suggestions on positioning, when pain medication worked best, and how to promote sleep for them both. I doubt that I would have had the opportunity to do this if they had not identified me, a nurse, as the person who could change dressings. Sometimes meeting the immediate need (often medically associated) gives the nurse the access to provide a full range of professional services.

Nursing activities can look like medical ones (although usually the similarity ends in the data gathering stage, and the therapeutic scope is different for both) and also can resemble "the same thing" as that provided by nonprofessional care-givers. However, the professional initiates the regimes, is accountable for the outcome, uses the access for a full range of services, and utilizes time during technical procedures to evaluate the client's total health functioning. Although the close affiliation with medicine has blurred the edge of discrete nursing practice, it has provided us the opportunity for the fullest and most accountable practice. Persons in need of nursing most often identify it in terms of sickness, not health. Since health has no broadly accepted boundaries, it is difficult to know when one's health is slipping or is not optimum. People are better able to define the sick role, and in seeking help to relieve illness, clients come into contact with nursing as an adjunct of medicine.

Many illnesses are the cause of unhealthful responses that autonomous nursing can resolve—another reason for the continuing close alliance of nursing and medicine. Illnesses can be resolved to the point of being cured and only at risk; such persons then come within the scope of nursing care, where proper preventive care and education can maintain health. Many of the problems that autonomous nursing practice is best equipped to solve often are directly attributable to the illness or sick role, such as immobility, malnutrition, pain, anxiety, noncompliance, depression, and skin breakdown.

The continuum between pathology and health is one with no dividing line at the midpoint. The extremes are determined easily, and separating nursing and medical accountability is reliable for both ends of the continuum. In the middle, however, where illness truly is at risk (even if absent), the convalescent is in need of medical supervision so nursing and medicine must maintain a close alliance. Even a healthy individual, confidently at the health end of this spectrum, can be catapulted quickly into the other end of the picture and in need of direct medical care. Nursing and medicine need each other to provide the best and most appropriate health care. The need for nursing to find an identity cannot compromise the need for closeness with medicine. Autonomy does not mean isolation. What will and should change in the future, however, is the separate identification of and reimbursement for nursing services.

THE PROBLEM OF ACCESS TO CLIENTS

The second reason for nursing's late blooming as a profession is that practitioners are primarily in employee positions and rarely have direct access to clients. The most legitimate employee status for any professional is to be hired by the person served. That client should have the opportunity to choose the professional and the services and to pay directly for the services. When someone other than the client does the hiring and paying, the individual's best interests are not always served. People value what they choose and contract for. Commitment to an individual care-giver always is more productive in terms of motivation and compliance than commitment to an organizational plan. When a client participates in setting health goals, and has a nurse also accountable for that activity (rather than the nurse's being accountable for organizational productivity), the client then receives truly professional care.

If punctuality, clean rooms, and quiet, content clients are the institution's goals, then nurse employees generally will try to achieve these—or resign. There is no opportunity in such a setting to have a nurse who will work flexible hours or be unconscious of mussed sheets, but who can goad and motivate and move a difficult patient toward health. One reason nurses become employees rather than go it alone is because they cannot articulate the range of professional therapies that differentiates them from other health care providers and therefore find it difficult to identify the services for which they should be sought out and paid. Another reason is that nursing has not recruited for the risk taker, the leader, the individual who is oriented to outcome and accomplishment. Rather, nursing has become a comfortable place for the occupational follower whose work is to be available for certain hours or shifts, who readily follows directions and orders, and who enjoys the hierarchy and the anonymity of uniforms.

Uniforms often are the last line of defense for the individual unsure of what the professional service is that makes nursing unique for clients. Without the uniform, perhaps the nurse would be indistinguishable from the nurse's aide. Unless nurses can voice the rationale and outcome of their actions, those functions may indeed be the same things as those of the aide. Uniforms, by representing a professional at work, often have become an empty symbol and a deception to clients. Better to abolish uniforms and depend on performance for identification of the professional at work.

When nurses are employees, patients cannot go directly to them for the resolution of health problems—the physician remains the gatekeeper to health care. This tends to reinforce the idea that nurses do not solve· primary problems. The existing employee status and secondary access will change only when the problems that nursing solves autonomously, and the special therapies that are used, are identified. The diagnosis and therapies must be spelled out in legislation that provides for direct reimbursement to nurses, and they will be used by nurses in informing clients what services to seek and expect from a professional.

Another way of differentiating between nursing and medical practice is to determine which of the two professionals is the primary therapist at any given stage of the client's health. When someone is ill, a physician is the legitimate therapist directing care. The nursing therapy during this period is primarily dependent and access is through the physician. As the client recuperates and reaches a state of resolving pathology but of high risk for recurrence, relapse, or other pathology, the direction of therapy is shared between nurse and physician. As the client reaches more stability, the director of therapy becomes the nurse. In regaining equilibrium, the client may identify, with the nurse, a level of health above what the person then enjoyed or had before the illness. The achievement of that more optimum state, or more low-risk stability, is the peak of nursing's autonomous activity.

Unfortunately, clients rarely are motivated to seek out knowledge and guidance in self-care or optimal health achievement until they are threatened by or experience illness. We in the nursing profession must assume some of the blame for this deficit in health care, for we have not made a concerted effort to assume leadership or to provide the knowledge and care needed for higher health status as the client's advocate and principal for health promotion.

THE PROBLEMS OF REIMBURSEMENT

Efforts to obtain direct payment and third party reimbursement must be preceded by articulating and demonstrating the unique and valuable services of professional nursing. An easier route for reimbursement and identity is to demonstrate the medical extender services that nurse practitioners are providing safely and effectively. The danger in this is that medical services will have been expanded without realization of the value of autonomous nursing service and the resulting demand for and use of health-promoting services. Autonomous nursing care is not a nurse's providing medical care without medical supervision; it is a nurse's providing nursing therapy that complements and often overlaps medical care.

THE EVOLVING ROLE OF NURSING EDUCATION

An important change that is occurring already in nursing is in the educational system. Most nurses have learned through an apprenticeship rather than an internship. An apprentice relies on copying the art of an acknowledged expert in the field. By doing what the expert does, the apprentice supposedly is duplicating the practice. An internship refers to a method of learning, during or after the formal educational program, where duplicating the thinking and decision-making patterns of an expert practitioner are mastered. Knowing the why and when of what to do are the hallmarks of such an experience. Knowing how, and duplicating that art successfully, also is a necessary component.

Since nursing is more than a visible craft and necessarily involves other human beings in the practice of the art, apprentices must learn when and why specific actions are taken. These actions relate primarily to medically directed nursing services—those that are curative and comfort oriented according to the pathology being treated. It is not surprising that the apprenticeship concept has sufficed for so long. When a person is accountable for doing what someone else has decreed, being expert only in the doing is enough. Being expert in actions is valuable and necessary in nursing—without it, the individual is left with a theory and no practice, which is not a profession. But practice without theory is nonprofessional, too. Many of the medically directed nursing activities learned as an apprentice to carry out medically directed care are the same actions as those used in a variety of autonomous nursing therapies. Nursing is prostituted when its practitioners learn primarily the actions of nursing in a framework of dependent, medically directed nursing care. Clients are cheated for the same reasons, for they receive only the potentiation of medical care, and true nursing care becomes a euphemism.

The rationale for nursing actions is provided in an apprenticeship education, but rarely to the extent that it is in an internship type of program. The internship program also provides the framework for two other aspects of professional nursing:

1. Many of the nursing activities used so effectively for medically directed care are visibly the same as those used autonomously by nurses to resolve health problems for their clients. Nurses in an internship program learn the full complement of situations in which to use their skilled actions—both autonomous and dependent.

2. Nurses learn how to incorporate theory fully into their practice by asking themselves not only "for what purpose" but also "for what outcome." In simplistic terms, an internship experience is designed for supervised decision making and evaluation of results as well as for developing mastery of skills.

The educational system is changing. The internship model soon will be the only one preparing professional nurses. A change in attitude about practice also is becoming apparent that at first seems antithetical to the move toward theory-based decision-making practice. As theory and decision-making abilities become more important in nursing education, the focus on practice as the ultimate goal has gained stature. In the past, the best nurses historically gravitated to supervising or teaching positions. Now rewards, both in prestige and in financial gain, are possible for master practitioners as well, and more of the best nurses are staying in the practice setting, demonstrating professional excellence that blends theory and skill. Before this major change, nursing educated its members by teaching appropriate actions and then promoting its best practitioners to supervisory positions. Nursing today has found a more appropriate reward for excellent practice and is beginning to recognize that leadership does not mean developing a hierarchy of order givers but rather providing the climate and support for each professional to carry out individual, autonomous services for clients.

For example, nursing leadership (at either the team leader or director of nursing level) was concerned with assigning tasks and monitoring their completion (for the team leader: baths, dressings, medications; for the director: staffing patterns, budget, inservice education). This obsession with process activities is changing and the focus is turning more toward goal achievement. The nursing leader is far more interested in helping practitioners develop health goals with their clients, by obtaining support for money, access, time, and tools, and by guiding these professionals in priority and goal setting. Just as nursing is actualization of a person's health potential, so is nursing leadership the potentiation of a nurse's best abilities. Nursing leadership means to nurse the nurse.

PROFESSIONALISM AND NURSING

No professionals take direction from their peers in how to carry out their activities. This is unacceptable in a true profession. It also is unethical if decision making regarding client health is vested in a nurse who does not have the professional training to be accountable for such freedom. Therefore, where practitioners are educated primarily in activities and not outcome, it is appropriate for nursing leadership to provide direction in how to go about these activities. Ethical safe practice for clients demands that only the fully prepared nurse has the freedom and responsibility to initiate and carry out an autonomous health plan.

Nursing's professional practice has been defined in New York State's Nurse Practice Act of 1972, and in many other states since then, as "diagnosing and treating human responses."[5] Responses change much more rapidly and more fluidly than pathology. For instance, the client who suffers a myocardial infarction has a clear medical problem. It will be with that person for a while. It is easy to focus on. It has discrete and measurable signs, symptoms, and evidence of progress. Electrocardiogram tracings and laboratory reports give credence to the pathology and to the course of the illness. This same client has important needs that we professional nurses can address, but the individual may not acknowledge those problems (depression, anxiety, fear of loss of sexual ability, threatened self-image, overdependence, overindependence) as readily, and the responses may flow between one and another as different goals are reached, thereby obliterating, for most purposes, the very goal achievement that supports nursing's unique worth.

For example, a heart attack victim who experiences and reports pain identifies a response amenable to nursing therapy. Analgesics, positioning, decreasing muscle tenseness through body contact, and counseling all can resolve the pain. However, as it recedes, the client's concerns may become those of anxiety and overdependence that then can become fear of loss of sexual ability and resulting overindependence. Each of these unhealthful responses may be resolved temporarily or permanently by nursing therapy. However, instead of a high sense of accomplishment by the nurse, and acknowledgment by the client, there often is only a change in focus and renewed efforts for equilibrium and comfort.

One nurse wrestling with this problem described a frustrating experience to me. She visited a client at home, specifically to address "persistent leg pains." The client was a bedridden woman, chronically ill and with numerous family problems. The nurse was able to alleviate the leg pain quickly by positioning (the woman was lying with her legs crossed and was unaware of her position). The woman then began to share her worries about her daughter, a teenager of particularly liberal social and sexual activity. They talked about ways of developing the girl's responsibility and maturity. Just when the nurse was sure the visit finally had centered on the woman's real need for nursing, the client burst into tears and wept bitterly about her feeling of utter uselessness. She had spoken in two hours of three different problems and yet at the end of the visit had totally confused the nurse as to which was the real health problem and what symptoms simply were masquerading as signs of other problems.

It is interesting to note that again and again clients will seek out a nurse for physical needs (leg pain) and use that access for more important help. If, as in this case, resolving a given unhealthful response only accommodates the identifying of another unhealthful response, there is no feeling of relief, accomplishment, or fulfillment. Maslow, Erikson,[6] and others believe a hierarchy of needs and development is necessary for the highest level of self-actualization, but the progression and dynamics of this process greatly hinder the evolution of lasting, identifiable health results through nursing therapy.

Rarely do clients see nursing results as exotic, exciting, and worthy of praise because nursing is enhancement and realization of self-care and optimum health. A simple extension of what one could do for oneself (if one were able, motivated, and visionary enough) is hardly worthy of applause as a unique and special service. Often the nature of the problem is that it cannot be acknowledged by the client, who therefore cannot acknowledge its successful resolution. For instance, either overdependence or overindependence may be inherently "O.K." behavior at a given time in a client's view. All the negative emotions (shame, anger, depression, anxiety) seem justified in the eyes of the person experiencing them. Therefore, the individual may not seek help to overcome them or thank the nurse who resolves them. Many may engage in unhealthful behavior at times and their defenses may preclude acknowledging the resolution. This is very unlike the practice of medicine, where the difficulties are voiced more readily and the treatment is more valued, welcomed, and identifiable. Only occasionally do individuals see the pathology as a negative reflection of themselves.

The easier it is to prove the existence of a problem, the easier it is to begin the appropriate treatment. Nursing suffers from a lack of discrete problem definition and predictable actions that clients can identify as therapies. Problem definition is becoming more definitive in nursing practice (see chapter 3 on diagnosis) but the actions that are therapies will continue to be mainly those other professionals and nonprofessionals use—teaching, diet prescription, toileting, ambulating, skin care, counseling, and exercising. The difference will be, as it is now, in the choice of appropriate predictable actions to accomplish stated health goals that were absent before the intervention began.

Nursing probably will adopt some of the so-called medical tools and processes (laboratory studies, x-ray) but the major components of practice will remain unique and more identifiable in outcome than in process.

It is becoming clearer what problems nursing resolves (diagnoses) and the states of health achievable (goals). What is still elusive is the therapy—actions alone or in combination—that are effective in all kinds of situations in preventing, maintaining, or promoting certain responses. The list of therapies is meager, unexciting, and shared with others. The excitement comes only when we nurses can say when we use the activities we are familiar with and what we can accomplish in a variety of circumstances.

Although these barriers remain to inhibit full identification of nursing as a profession, we must continue the work of defining and providing what it is that clients need that no other profession does as well—that mysterious element called professional nursing practice.

NOTES

1. Catherine M. Norris, "Direct Access to the Patient," *American Journal of Nursing,* May 1970, p. 1010.

2. Nancy S. Keller, "The Nurse's Shrinking Role: Is It Expanding or Shrinking?" *Nursing Outlook,* April 1973, Vol. 21, No. 4, p. 236.

3. M. Lucille Kinlein, *Independent Nursing Practice with Clients* (Philadelphia: J. B. Lippincott Co., 1977), p. 117.

4. Anna B. Dugan, "Nursing Autonomy: Key to Quality Nurturance," *Journal of Nursing Administration,* July-August 1971, p. 51.

5. New York State Nurse Practice Act, 1972.

6. Erik H. Erikson, *Childhood and Society* (New York: W. W. Norton and Co., 1950), p. 269.

Chapter 2

Catchwords for Nursing

In the last few years a number of words have become entrenched in nursing literature and have been used with such repetition as to become almost a litany. Although dictionaries define their meanings for general use, the nuances the words have assumed in defining the professional practice of nursing have not been explored thoroughly.

The words we nurses use to define ourselves and our relationships are important indicators of our self-awareness as developing professionals and of our expectations of relationships with other health care workers and with our clients.

Some of the words lack clear meanings even for those in nursing, which will continue to confuse both colleagues and clients. If a consensus can be reached on the discrete meanings and expectations inherent in these descriptive catchwords, perhaps that can be a strong basis for defining clearly to others what nursing service and relationships should be. This searching to define ourselves is part of the politics of nursing's survival. Nurses too long have been defined by others, often to fill in the missing (or undervalued) aspects of another service such as medical, social, or environmental. Clients need to know how we nurses define ourselves and our service if they are to know what to seek us out for; coprofessionals need to know how to complement or supplement each other. That is where words and clear definitions enter the picture to help clarify actual or potential misunderstandings.

Each group of words discussed here has similar generic meanings but specifically suggests different expectations and relationships. All dictionary meanings are quoted from *The Random House Dictionary of the English Language,* unabridged edition (1966), or *The Random House College Dictionary* (1975).

19

AUTONOMY VS. INDEPENDENCE

Autonomous: "self-governing; independent; subject to its own laws only."

Independent: "not influenced or controlled by others in matters of opinion, conduct, etc.; thinking or acting for oneself." "not subject to another's authority or jurisdiction; autonomous; free." "possessing a competency."

The core of autonomous practice is being able to offer a unique therapy. Not as central, but just as necessary, is the freedom to provide that service without interference or permission.

Autonomous and independent are similar in meaning and both have a sense of being free from something. Both describe that freedom in terms of absence of other influence or control rather than in terms of something to be free from. Most acknowledged professions do not make an issue of their autonomy. Most have had no need to. In the case of nursing, the autonomy or independence is indeed a freeing from the boundary of dependent medical practice. It must mean that nurses are free to do something different, something more, than before. Our work still may encompass some medically directed activities, but autonomous practice demands that there be elements of theory and practice unique to the nursing profession and directed, initiated, and performed by nurses. When we have knowledge and skill equal to those who heretofore directed us, then we can share in initiating those activities in the future.

This means that many activities, both past and current, that nurses perform only under the direction or supervision of another professional (usually medical) may become elements of autonomous nursing practice when the knowledge of why, as well as how, becomes part of our repertoire.

Although the two words may seem to mean the same thing, antonomous may say it better because of the phrase "subject to its own laws only." This seems to be the one acknowledgment that there is matter involved in what nurses are free to do, and without that special content, we are not legitimately autonomous or independent.

Therapy: "The treatment of disease, as by some remedial or curative process. A curative power or quality." From the Greek therapeia = healing

Care: "to be concerned or solicitous. To watch over. To act on, deal with, attend to."

Intervention: "To come between, intercede. To occur . . . to modify or hinder."

Practice: "The exercise or pursuit of a profession. Repeated performance."

Therapy is a special kind of activity that makes an undesirable condition better, or prevents it from occurring. It is a "special" kind of care in that it is theory-based; it is provided by a professional practitioner. Professional *practice* is the comprehensive activity of diagnosing, goal setting, planning, giving, and evaluating care. Therapy is a component of professional practice; it is the care for problem resolution or problem prevention. Whenever professionals use their distinct skills to resolve or prevent an undesirable (usually unhealthful) condition, those activities are therapy. There are medical therapy, physical therapy, mental therapy, occupational therapy . . . and nursing therapy. There is also educational therapy when something in the individual learning process goes wrong, and legal therapy when legal steps can remove someone from jeopardy or harm. Obviously, educational or legal *practice* involve far more than the therapeutic steps, and there can be no therapy without the total professional practice of which it is a component. Therapeutic (making better or less in danger) activities can be carried on by many, but the therapy and its direction and the protocol of diagnosis, alternative plans, care, and the resulting evaluation, come from a professional. Without this methodical and accountable framework, the helpful activities are simply care, not therapy.

Some therapies are interventions—stopping or interceding in a set of events that are unhealthful. Intervention usually means cutting a link or removing something problematical. It doesn't have an additive connotation, which is sometimes part of therapy. Therapy usually signifies professional activity designed for an individual's benefit—the client's. (Therapy is not always restorative as identified in medicine.) It can be activity-aimed at preserving the status quo, which might be at risk, or aimed at strengthening a useful client activity (exercise or diet compliance).

It is a generic professional term and it "belongs" in nursing just as it belongs as part of any professional practice. The content differs, and that is necessary in order to differentiate nursing from other professions. It is very much related to diagnosis; one is the identification of a problem requiring attention, and therapy is that problem-specific resolution.

EXPANDED ROLE AND EXTENDED PRACTICE

Expanded: "increased in area, bulk or volume; enlarged."

Extended: "stretched out." "increased length or duration."

The nurse practitioner role, which generally means providing primary care using physical assessment and history-taking skills, often has been described as the expanded or extended practice of nursing. Early writing on the subject interchanged the two. Expanded has a multidimentional sense to it. It may mean new methods and a new outcome. Extended is more unidirectional, more oriented toward meeting a predetermined goal. For instance, expanded practice might mean that the limits of what might occur are open and unknown—that nurses have added new tools and where those tools will take us is as yet unknown. Extended practice may mean growth in one dimension only, such as using the same tools and the same outcome but moving into a new area, such as from inpatient to outpatient care.

Many nurses feel that the new skills of physical assessment and history taking are simply a fuller complement (extension) of our already developed data gathering ability—that we will continue to make diagnoses within the realm of nursing and that the scope of our services is the same, but that we have more complete primary data with which to work.

Others feel that the new skills will open new areas of diagnosis and therapy and that nursing service will expand.

Many in nursing believe that our skills and therapy are broadening as are all professional fields of practice. When physicians learned new therapies such as joint replacement, cardiac bypass techniques, or hyperalimentation, these were not defined as expanding or extending their role. If nursing's growth is regarded in analogous terms, perhaps that growing service is not extended or expanded practice but rather the natural and desired thrust of progress seen in any true professional group. What makes the analogy fuzzy, though, is that these new skills already are practiced by an existing group (physicians).

Some nurses see the new tools of physical assessment and history taking and the new emphasis on identifiable clients and a measurable outcome as natural growths of their profession. They are filling the new framework with nursing content and would like to forget the expanded or extended labels. Others who are using the history-taking and physical assessment skills to provide medical care may indeed be practicing in an extended or expanded role. If the therapy no longer is nursing therapy but a tangential medical therapy, then a label probably is appropriate. But this is an extension of the dependent nursing role, not the autonomous or professional role.

COLLABORATION: COOPERATION COME OF AGE

Collaborate: "to work, one with another."

Cooperate: "to work or act together or jointly for a common purpose or benefit, to provide more or less active assistance."

Although the dictionary meanings are nearly identical for these two words, there are some hints at the widening difference. "Assistance" is a different level of autonomy than "working one with another." Assistance suggests that someone else is providing the direction and the leadership. Working one with another suggests more teamwork and a dual role. Operationally the two words have continued to develop differently, especially in professional circles, where coprofessional relationships are being redefined.

The vital difference between these words is the sense of equality in collaboration and of compromise in cooperation. For most of their professional lives, nurses have been only too ready to cooperate, mostly with physicians and administrators. If their personal characteristics were enumerated, cooperation probably would be near the top. Nurses have been the followers in most decisions affecting patient care. Nurses needed only to hear that it would be better for the patient and they willingly would work harder, longer, more blindly, and for less money. Cooperate has the sense of going along with one's superior (parent, teacher, boss). One cooperates; one doesn't cause trouble. Cooperate has a sense of giving up one's own beliefs or methods in order to effect another (more powerful, more persuasive?) viewpoint or goal. Cooperation does not seem to require any autonomous action; indeed that might get in the way of cooperation. There also is the feeling that the other goal could not be achieved without that assistance.

Collaboration, on the other hand, is cooperation come of age. It means equal cooperation in goal setting and in action. Collaboration is enhancing teamwork. It is responsible cooperation among equals that results in more than the two could do alone. It is cooperation without compromise. To read the literature, it might be thought that nurses were involved everywhere in the strongest of collaborative arrangements. Not so. Collaboration may be an idea whose time has not yet come. True collaboration means acknowledgment by all parties that there is indeed the potential for equal input, equal leadership, and equal value. Nursing is on the brink of demonstrating that fact, but until it is accepted by nurses and our fellow collaborators, we are only cooperating under the guise of collaboration. Surely nurses can chuckle at the innocent secondary dictionary meaning of collaboration as cooperating with the enemy. The primary meaning, "to work, one with another" has great promise for their work. Collaboration may be the strongest means of providing nursing's unique yet subtle service: collaboration with physicians, clients, and most of all, with our fellow nurses.

ACCOUNTABLE: THE WORD WITH THE TWO-WAY SOUND

Accountable: "subject to having to report, explain or justify; responsible; answerable."

Responsible: "answerable or accountable, as for something within one's power, control, or management," "having a capacity for moral decisions and therefore accountable; capable of rational thought or action."

Responsibility means that someone has been directed, or is expected, to do something (or not to do something). It usually has to do with actions. There also is a general feeling that the word means someone is telling another someone that he or she is responsible. There is a sense of direction involved in responsible. Responsible says one goes about something in the right way. It is a very process-oriented word.

Accountable is different in two ways. It means answerable, which is, so to speak, after the fact. It also has the sense of outcome accomplishment rather than process. People are more likely to say accountable when they are looking for justification for an outcome, whereas responsible is used more often when describing an action to be carried out. Nurses have felt responsibility in our profession for a long time, mostly for those regimes promoted by our superiors. Accountable, especially for outcome and not just process, is new to the profession and is more likely to be used in context with autonomous practice.

In many ways all of these word differences are similar to cooperate and collaborate. Both collaboration and accountability are hallmarks of professional interactions; cooperation and responsibility are more descriptive of dependent functioning. Accountable also is far more apt in describing interrelationships with a client than is responsible. Accountable has a two-way sound about it.

Two different professionals (a nurse and a physician) with the same client (or different clients) can be responsible for the same things (in terms of initiation and methodology), but because of different and unique theory and therapy, they will be accountable for different results.

CLIENT—SUCCESSOR TO PASSIVE PATIENT

Client: "anyone under the patronage of another; a dependent." "a person who is receiving the benefits, services, etc., of a (social welfare agency, a government bureau, etc.).” “A person who applies . . . for advice or commits his cause to management.”

Patient: “a person or thing that undergoes some action.” archaic: “sufferer or victim.” Syn: invalid.

The word patient in the traditional medical system connotes passiveness: the patient is diagnosed, treated, and given prescriptions and orders for therapy. The word client does not have this passive connotation.

> In the nursing relationship, the client is active: he seeks the help of the nurse, and part of the nursing care that is given is helping the client to recognize and communicate his needs. The client must, in my concept of nursing, be active. He asks questions and receives full answers; he takes an active part as we assess his self-care ability and as we initiate improvements. Thus, the word “client” seems to be appropriate in conveying many important aspects of my nursing practice.[1]

That says it well. The dictionary has a few other distinguishing characteristics between the words. Most of those who agree on the passive/active difference still would be surprised at how narrowly the word patient is defined in the dictionary. Not only does it label patient as a sufferer or victim but it also gives invalid as the synonym.

The meaning of client is more wide ranging and active. Client is of the same genre as collaborative and accountable. The client is a necessary decision-making partner in the system this word definition process is identifying.

THE ROLES OF ASSISTANT AND ASSOCIATE

Assistant: “serving in an immediately subordinate position; having secondary rank.”

Associate: “connected, joined, or related, esp. as a companion or colleague; having equal or nearly equal responsibility.”

The differences between these two words are well known. What is particularly interesting is how pejorative sounding the dictionary description of assistant is. Most nurses have spent years being proud and gaining

status by assisting physicians. Now the dictionary tells us that a second
rate role is that of an assistant. In gaining associate status, it is to be hoped
that nursing does not sell out the valuable and gratifying actions of
assistant. Autonomous practice is the most complete and most professional
role in nursing. Without autonomy, nursing becomes a service directed by
someone else, and is at risk for being limited to those things known and
valued by that director. "Professional" includes autonomy, and with that
free-standing authority comes the full scope of nursing service. What must
be remembered however, is that those services requiring nursing autonomy
(identifying and resolving health problems such as anxiety or noncompliance for instance) are not always the services currently most important
to a client. In other words, a nurse with the professional and autonomous
skills in resolving anxiety or noncompliance may be most valuable to a
critically ill person by providing not the comprehensive skills listed above,
but providing positioning, suctioning, and bathing. If, in developing the
professional aspects of nursing, we were to overstate their constant value
over the technical aspects of nursing we would be wrong. If technical
nursing were to die to allow professional nursing to flourish, everyone
would be the losers. Being an associate means sharing not only responsibility but also many of the activities. Associate is a word related to peer
and to colleague.

COLLEAGUE, PEER, UNIQUE, EXPERT, EQUAL

Colleague: "an associate in an office, profession, work."
Peer: "a person of the same rank or standing; a legal
equal." "a person who is equal to another in
abilities, qualifications, etc."
Unique: "having no like or equal." "limited in occurrence
to a given class." "The only specimen of a given
kind." "impossible to duplicate within a stated or
implied scope."
Expert: "a person who has special skill or knowledge in
some particular field." "authority." "possessing special skill or knowledge; trained by practice."
Equal: "as great as." "like or alike in quantity, degree,
value."

Colleague and peer have a nice collaborative sound. A colleague for a
nurse is another nurse, someone who shares one's profession. Colleague
usually is associated with the professions; the more technical occupations

will have coworkers instead. Whereas colleagues are within a profession, peers are from different professions but hold equal status or rank. Peers relate laterally. Being a peer makes collaboration much more likely and requires acknowledgment by both participants of peer standing.

An individual does not decide unilaterally on peer or colleague standing, although colleague probably is reached more objectively since it involves credentials that are the same as someone else's. A nurse is a nurse is a nurse, but is a nurse equal to a physician? Peer standing requires that both groups acknowledge their equal footing. It means nothing if nurses tell physicians they are peers and the physicians do not also acknowledge the nurses as their peers.

It can be an easy thing to claim a peer relationship, but this is a reciprocal position. In Shakespeare's *King Henry IV,* Part I, an interchange between Glendower and Hotspur makes this clear:

Glendower: I can call spirits from the vasty deep.
Hotspur: Why, so can I, or so can any man;
            But will they come when you do call for them?

Unique means having no like or equal. It also means, in professional parlance, that one has or does something different, unusual, and special. Equal can mean two things: doing the same thing, or doing different things of the same value. A service can be both unique and equal; unique in having components shared by no one else, and yet being equal with other services in value and autonomy. If a unique theory base and practice are truly discriminating factors in determining a profession, then it can be said that possessing uniqueness gives an individual a component of being equal in worth, or service, to another different (unique) professional. Of course, this does not make for exact equals, but rather equals in terms of each person's being a professional. It means being as great as.

So, for redirection in this word maze, for nurses to be considered as an equal or a peer by physicians and clients, there must be a unique theory-practice base. This is a hallmark of the professions and helps justify nursing's legitimate claim to peer standing in the health professions.

Many physicians and clients have long acknowledged that nursing holds equal importance or value with medicine but only in that it offers a necessary extension of medical services. Without the unique and equal nurse-physician standing (true peer relationship), clients are at risk for receiving only medical care and not the needed complement of professional nursing care.

Expertness has a special meaning for the professions. A unique theory-practice base is necessary for every profession. Since expert is defined as "special skill or knowledge; trained by practice," the role is very close to professional. But is every professional an expert or does expertness happen within a profession? Is every nurse an expert in nursing? Certainly a professional nurse has special skill and/or knowledge. Being trained by practice is part of becoming a nurse. But does acquiring special skill and knowledge and being trained by practice make one an expert?

An expert is one who knows why and how and also is a master practitioner who performs a craft in the best possible way. Therefore, not every member of a professional group is an expert in the sense of performing in an optimal way, but only the members of that profession can be the experts.

For a long time nursing was viewed as a medically directed practice. When and what nurses did for clients was decided and ordered by physicians, who often determined in part how it was done as well. But there also was a strong consensus among nurses and physicians that nurses were the experts at delivering or performing nursing care. That meant that the bathing, positioning, and physical care components were performed most expertly by nurses. So in a time when nursing was seen solely as an arm of medicine, the practice component of nursing was identified as expertness.

As the theory base from which nursing practice is derived is identified and broadened, the expertness of deciding when and what nursing care should be provided also is being acknowledged. For example, if nurses are the experts in positioning, then we also should direct when and for what purpose this function should be performed. If the medical problem (such as multiple fractures) were a factor in positioning, then nursing and medicine would have to share their expertness in determining a positioning plan. If positioning is for a nursing problem (potential contractures following a stroke, for example) then nurses are the experts and can implement their regime autonomously. Expertness is another component of determining peer standing. A profession must have a unique base as well as master (expert) practitioners.

FOUR DEFINITIONS ATTAINING LEGAL SIGNIFICANCE

Assessment: "act of . . . appraisal; evaluation." "to estimate or judge value or character."

Need: "a requirement." "a necessity." "a lack of something deemed necessary."

Problem: "any question or matter involving doubt, uncertainty/difficulty." "question proposed for solution."

Diagnose: "to ascertain the cause or nature of from the symptoms. To determine on the basis of scientific examination."

The differences, similarities, and confusions among these words have been noted and argued, but not resolved completely. Progress, however, is being made.

Nurse practice acts are being revised in every state. To gain acceptance for passage in state legislatures, much of the new language is being accompanied by a definition of terms. More and more, diagnosis is finding its discrete place in nursing's legal services. In defining diagnosis, the three other terms—need, problem, and assessment—must be differentiated clearly.

The process of assessment includes gathering data and determining which are useful in reaching a diagnosis and ordering and evaluating the facts in light of what is pertinent to the specific person's health status. A diagnosis is the end product of assessment, whereby a judgment is made as to what the specific deficit (if any) is and, if possible, the cause. A health deficit that nursing therapy can resolve is a nursing diagnosis. Problems usually exist as a result of an unmet need. To look at it another way: Everyone has needs, basic ones such as food, air, love, and shelter, as well as more individualized needs such as milk, moist air, sexual love, a private room of one's own, etc. When these needs or requirements are not being met, a problem exists. If such a problem involves a health deficit that nursing can resolve, it is a nursing diagnosis.

A diagnosis showing a health deficit related to an unmet need, for example, could be "extreme agitation related to lack of privacy" or "hacking cough related to breathing dry air." A diagnosis is a value judgment about what has gone wrong. It is based on a thorough gathering of data and an evaluation of those facts to determine which ones will suggest and validate the diagnosis.

There are, of course, nursing needs and nursing problems, too. Nursing needs are those elements required by nurses to provide care needed by the client. These needs include access, continuity of contact, freedom to prescribe and act, and feedback from the client and other care givers. Nursing problems are those that interfere with meeting nursing needs; for example, limited access, rotating case load, unavailability of data, or inadequate time.

The difference between problem and diagnosis is seen less easily. A problem is an unsatisfactory condition requiring resolution in order to meet a need. Problems can be self-identified or professionally identified.

They may be self-resolved or by others or even by time or chance. Some problems are not related to health (they may be financial or learning, for instance) and in fact the resolution of some problems may result in a more unhealthful state. For example, a woman with chronic renal disease has trouble becoming pregnant; when her fertility problem is solved, she may become acutely ill and even die.

Problems, then, are not necessarily nursing diagnoses. Nursing diagnoses are special kinds of problems—health deficits identified by and treated by nurses. Clients obviously can identify some of their own nursing diagnoses. Most of these cannot be resolved without the client's positive participation. But it is the necessary nursing guidance and/or therapy that makes the identification of specific problems nursing diagnoses (see Figure 2-1).

Another difference is that nursing diagnostic statements are a result of professional inference concerning both the problem and its cause. Problem statements, by comparison, are more general and factual, and do not always identify the cause.

Part of nurses' identity is determined by the way we describe ourselves in the language we share with other health professionals. We are coming late to this full identity, and others already have laid claim to the words and to their own uniqueness in health care. We have a particularly challenging job in redefining ourselves. Springing afresh on the health care scene might be easier than changing the image of nursing's medically

---

Figure 2-1   Nursing Diagnosis of Health Needs

health needs

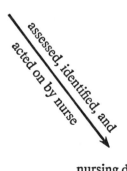

health problems

nursing diagnoses

dependent practice to one that also encompasses its own uniqueness. Proper use of words can help tell that story.

Nurses need to be together on the words we use to describe our special service. We need to spread the word about nursing so that our clients will know what nurses have to offer and where we fit in the health care system that serves them. Alice in *Alice's Adventures in Wonderland* shared this problem.[2]

> "Then you should say what you mean," the March Hare went on.
>
> "I do," Alice hastily replied; "at least—at least I mean what I say—that's the same thing, you know."
>
> "Not the same thing a bit!" said the Hatter. "Why, you might just as well say that 'I see what I eat' is the same thing as 'I eat what I see'!"

It will be better for nursing if we follow the Hare's advice. Surely we always have been sincere, which is Alice's plea. But being sincere isn't enough. Now it is time to be precise. And strong.

NOTES

1. M. Lucille Kinlein, R.N., *Independent Nursing Practice With Clients* (Philadelphia: J. B. Lippincott Co., 1977), p. 8.

2. Lewis Carroll, *Alice's Adventures In Wonderland* (N.Y.: Rainbow Classics, World Press, 1946), p. 75.

SUGGESTED READING

Block, Doris. "Some Crucial Terms in Nursing: What Do They Really Mean?" *Nursing Outlook,* November 1974, p. 689.

——————— *The Expanded Role of The Nurse,* Contemporary Nursing Series (N.Y.: Ed. Services Div., AJN Co., 1973).

Mundinger, Mary, and Jauron, Grace. "Developing a Nursing Diagnosis." *Nursing Outlook,* February 1975, p. 94.

Vincent, Pauline. "Some Crucial Terms in Nursing—A Second Opinion." *Nursing Outlook,* January 1975, p. 46.

Chapter 3

The Nursing Process: Problem Solving for Health

"The nursing process sounds like a lot of work. It sounds dry, stuffy, analytical and certainly not very action oriented. I hardly have enough time now to do what I have to do. How can I add this time-consuming task to my day?"

Analytical yes, time-consuming yes, but the kind of nursing care that is the end result may take less time than the rituals so readily implemented without benefit of an analytical problem-solving process. The process clearly provides solid assistance in giving nursing care. This chapter analyzes the process in two segments, the first a fairly concise rundown of a six-step guideline, then a detailed expansion of those points, including numerous examples.

The way nurses go about their work, the results achieved, and the expectations of client participation in care all come together in the nursing process. Other disciplines use the same problem-solving process; only the content differs.

The nursing process in various forms has been in the literature for years. Most often it is described as a three-part process of assessment, implementation, and evaluation. Assessment has meant many things to many people. Most often it encompasses the data gathering and problem identification steps. Sometimes it also includes goal setting and planning. Agreement still has not been reached on its components of assessment. When use of the term is so poorly standardized, expectations in practice vary and practitioners are confused in communicating about the first phase of planning care for clients.

The implementation phase will be incomplete and not as clear or predictable as it should be unless that step is a direct result of assessment and planning. Implementation can mean performing the activities dictated by institutional policy ("vital signs will be taken twice a day unless otherwise ordered," "preop patients will be NPO (Nothing By Mouth) after midnight") or by physician's regimen ("dressing to incision site TID (Three Times a Day)", or "ambulate with assistance q. d. (every day)"). In both cases the implementation phase follows not the nursing assessment but the assessment or prediction of needs by another group or professional. Evaluation in this three-part fuzzy system rarely is carried out because there is a lack of consensus on what is being evaluated or who is accountable for that process. Again, with no agreement on definitions and expectations, there can be no consensus in practice. This consensus is required if nurses are to communicate effectively with one another about the kinds of problems their clients experience, the data that should be sought to validate discrete problem definition, the kinds of goal achievement that can be expected, and the nursing therapies that can reach those goals. This is the nursing process.

THE NEED FOR A COMMON TOOL

If nurses use different process models, the results and expectations will differ. More importantly, we will not be able to learn from one another about successful solving of problems nor be able to prescribe effective therapies on the basis of another's successful assessment work. There is a need to be able to exchange, use, and build on a body of workable and effective nursing therapy. That will come years sooner if we have a common tool to go about our work and to measure the effectiveness of our actions. That tool is the nursing process.

The nursing process has been called the helping process or the problem-solving process. It is used in its generic sense by all professionals for problem solving and therefore for helping.

A Common Denominator Process

Nursing uses the process in its basic sense—for problem solving. The component steps in the process also can be useful in specific ways. The process can identify the scope of the profession by testing problems nurses solve, data they need to elicit, goals they can assist clients in reaching, and therapies used to achieve those goals. Not only can nurses borrow from one another in identifying problems or appropriate goals and therapies, we also can begin to predict problems on the basis of common data and judge how much time is needed to accomplish goals in given circumstances. Only with the common denominator of a single kind of process can nurses effectively learn from each others' problem-solving work.

It is important for nurses to recognize the intellectual activities required in professional care. A good nurse historically has been measured from the neck down: busy hands and busy feet. A busy head more often than not was not valued or got in the way of other professionals who had taken the prerogative of nursing care planning as their own. Because giving care, rather than decision making and planning, has been the most rewarded activity in nursing, the process may seem to be an extra, the icing on the cake that may not be necessary and that certainly is not the priority ahead of doing. The process can make the doing more specific, problem resolving, and less ritualistic. It can cut down on the time spent giving care by eliminating activities the client does not really need and by truly individualizing care.

The Overbathing Syndrome and Time Saving

The process focuses on activities that are targeted for specific problem resolution. Therefore, the progress of that resolution will signal the change or cessation of activities that otherwise might go on (unproductively) for days.

For instance, much of nursing's ritualistic and time-consuming activities are in bathing. We somehow have accepted the idea that a daily case load of ten hospitalized clients means ten baths. Clean skin means less chance of infection and greater comfort; however, oversolicitious bathing actually can increase the chance of infection (dry and chafed skin) and decrease comfort (itching and flaking). Even frequent linen changes (with the fresh but often harsh linen) can increase skin chafing and irritation. On the other hand, in addition to cleanliness and comfort, bathing also may promote relaxation and sleep. For all of these reasons, only a few complete morning baths and bed changes should be planned, and others should be scheduled for evening hours; still others should not occur at all—thereby providing time for more needed nursing activities.

A SIX-STEP NURSING PROCESS AS GUIDELINE

The following definitive six-step process should be useful to nurses, who should:

1. diagnose the unhealthful problem and the etiology
2. identify data that validate the problem and examine for completeness
3. decide what goal can be reached in improving the health status or behavior

4. formulate a plan of nursing intervention, including referrals and joint efforts with others
5. implement the care process, make the referrals, and coordinate efforts
6. evaluate the effectiveness of the nursing intervention in resolving the diagnosis

Effective nursing care begins with the identification of the health problem to be treated—a nursing diagnosis that directs all the other nursing activities.

The Evolution of a Diagnosis

With that succinct overview of the nursing, the expanded analysis begins with the fact that making a diagnosis in any profession is a process of inferring a problem based on the available information. Although the information is what leads to the diagnosis, irrelevant data always are present. Therefore, identifying the data that specifically validate each individual health problem is a vital step following the diagnosis.

Identification of Validating Data

As the professional begins to determine a diagnosis, the next step is to examine available information and see whether everything needed is present. For instance, if a tentative diagnosis of "noncompliance with medical regimen" is being considered, the data needed include evidence of noncompliance (verbalized by client, or perhaps measurable data such as medication not taken as validated by unchanging number of pills in bottle). If the only evidence for noncompliance is an unchanging medical condition, there are other possibilities such as ineffective therapy or a new or undiagnosed illness.

The process of selecting the appropriate data from that available also tends to identify missing information that can make a specific diagnosis less likely. The difference between "fear of pain" and "pain" may be the reporting of pain by a client—the subjective finding. Objectively, the nurse might see the guarding, wincing, and withdrawal that go with both. However, without the report of experienced pain, the differentiation between pain and fear of pain cannot be made. The interventions for fear of pain and for pain also are different. Therefore, without the subjective information of experienced pain from the client, not enough data are available to make a definitive diagnosis.

The Establishment of Goals

Once the problem has been defined and validated by examining the data, the next step is determining what goal can be reached either to eliminate the health problem or to begin its resolution. The goal is a statement of a client's behavior ("client reports pain-free state 20 minutes after medication and positioning") that shows improvement from the original unhealthful response.

The Formulation of the Plan

Only when the goal is determined can the plan be formulated, because the plan's function is to assist the client in reaching that goal: the plan is not holistic, it is goal specific. It is a set of orders for nursing personnel to carry out. It should be specific as to how, where, when, and who ("give pain medication immediately on request if over three hours since last medication. Do not initiate other nursing activities until pain relief is obtained").

Implementation of the Care Process

The implementation of care is the actual carrying out of the activities and the documentation ("pain medication given on request; pain relief obtained within 15 minutes"). Obviously, much nursing care in hospitals—perhaps even the majority—is not related directly to meeting the goals set by client and nurse. The medically directed activities are the majority and they must be performed and documented. But these usually are part of routine (or medically directed care) and not part of the nursing process. In an ambulatory setting with nurse practitioners, the majority of the care will be directed by the nursing process.

The nursing process directs and measures effective problem-resolving care. It is not a method of providing comprehensive or holistic care. Focusing on resolving one problem or reaching one goal is far more effective and measurable than trying to do everything at once. This does not mean that a number of problem-resolving, goal-achieving plans cannot be implemented at the same time. In fact, a number of goals can be determined and listed separately in one comprehensive plan. The difficulty in this system is that it is difficult to determine which parts of the plan contributed to success or failure in the different goal achievements. This makes it unclear what to include in the plan when only one of the goals, at another time and for another client, is being addressed. For example:

1. client verbalizes pain-free state 20 minutes after medication
2. ambulates with assistance of only one person
3. demonstrates effective use of IPPB (Intermittent Positive Pressure Breathing) treatment

These are different goals that all may be reached through a plan of early pain medication followed by a 15-minute inactive period for the medication to begin working, followed by a comfortable ambulation (which may increase depth of respiration) and then IPPB practice.

The Final Phase: Evaluation

The final step in the nursing process is evaluation. It is the judgment about whether or not the nursing intervention was successful. Three major factors are responsible for the absence of this step in most nursing practice:

1. It is not always clear what is being evaluated. Is it problem resolution, goal achievement, or whether the plan was carried out? Any one can happen without the other.
2. Evaluation bears a definite succeed-fail label and precludes the failures' being fully addressed. Evaluation is far more useful if looked on as a judgment about what worked and why and what kinds of variables tend to impinge on success. It is necessary to erase the stigma of failure in nursing therapy, and instead to look at what factors promote or hinder goal achievement in different circumstances.
3. Part of the failures story is that there are so many variables that it is difficult and frustrating to isolate and evaluate the effectiveness of nursing interventions. However, the answers are so valuable and useful in planning nursing care that evaluation, although complex and often painful, should be attempted.

This six-step process, then, can be used definitively to solve health problems for clients and to document for the health care community as a whole the special process and outcomes of professional nursing service.

AUTONOMOUS NURSING FUNCTIONS ESSENTIAL

The process must include autonomous nursing functions to qualify as a method for planning professional care, even though the same process obviously can be used to plan dependent nursing care. Using the current medical diagnosis as the focus, whether or not curing disease is the goal, the supplemental nursing actions specific to resolving that pathology then could be written into the plan, carried out, and evaluated as part of the medical regimen's effectiveness. This complex and time-consuming process can be avoided simply by listing those dependent nursing functions in the medical regimen in the process of gathering data, diagnosing, and treating.

The nursing process, however, requires step-by-step development and documentation for many reasons. Most important, a diagnostic classification that provides labels, signs, and symptoms for the health problems that nurses diagnose and treat autonomously does not exist.

The kinds of nursing care required for medical diagnoses are better known and therefore more predictable and standardized than the therapies needed for nursing diagnoses. Efforts have been made to develop and publish protocols and standard nursing care plans that can be used with success with various medical diagnoses. By using these, nurses can save their creative care planning for the resolution of diagnoses where it is not yet known what works best.

Progress also is being made nationally in classifying nursing diagnoses and describing the signs and symptoms for each. More work is needed, particularly from practicing nurses, regarding the distinguishing characteristics of these nursing-specific health problems.

Goal setting, too, needs further development so that identification of health goals that really resolve unhealthful responses can be continued and reasonable estimates can be made about how long each goal will take to achieve and what the appropriate intermediate and terminal goals should be.

Planning the nursing actions that can achieve the goals is a key to effective practice: what nursing therapy is needed to raise a person's health status? This is where the ordinariness of so many nursing actions takes on clear importance. When it can be shown what those actions achieve—the back rub, the skillful positioning, specific teaching, and ambulation—all are seen in very different perspective if nurses can demonstrate what these therapies alone or in combination can accomplish. Implementing is the doing and documenting of planned nursing care. This, too, takes on greater meaning and accountability when related directly to problem resolution and goal achievement.

Evaluation, uncertain as it may be, provides the answers for modifying and improving care in future successful planning with clients. Evaluation is a judgment as to whether a given plan was effective in resolving the unhealthful response (nursing diagnosis).

In order to do this, two things must happen. First the nurse must determine whether the original unhealthful behavior has changed to healthier behavior. Second, the nurse must ascertain whether the plan was followed, because some unhealthful behavior may change without any intervention, and it would be a mistake to credit an inoperable plan with success.

Many would say, correctly, that problem definition, goal-directed activities, and evaluation of their effectiveness always have taken place in professional nursing care. However, the way problem definition was carried out in the past was vague and indefinite—either not written at all or written only in medical terms. Often the approach was by trial and error (also rarely written or communicated), which hardly ever was evaluated for effectiveness. Because historical data are lacking on how this process has been carried out intuitively for years, it is now necessary to develop the knowledge of effective nursing care so that it is written and linked systematically from data to diagnosis to goals to planning to implementing to evaluation. If this is not reduced to writing, knowledge for retrieval and future use will not be available. If the steps are not linked together, there will be no problem-specific therapy. For all their unrealistic and godlike aspirations to deliver "holistic" care, nurses have achieved little that is measurable or predictable. If we can be satisfied with a smaller, more discrete slice of health care, perhaps we can demonstrate our measurable and valuable service: solving identifiable health problems rather than trying to direct, coordinate, and give all care to all people.

COMPONENTS OF PREDICTABLE CARE

A written and systematic process is essential to scientifically predictable care. The other necessary component is identifiable, accountable, authoritative nursing care for every client. The models of practice that combine these elements are described in the chapters on Primary Nursing, Nurse Practitioner, and Community Nurse. Some nursing leaders have questioned whether theirs is indeed a profession since it seems to function without a theory and by trial and error. Others have said nursing theory exists but is difficult to identify because individual practitioners must seek it out in their observation of effective care. In other words, nursing is a practice in search of a theory. If nursing is indeed a theory-based profession, the nursing process can help identify that theory by showing what works for whom and in what circumstances to bring about healthier conditions. For those who believe that nursing activities are trial and error and that they have no basis in theory, the process can put the practice components in order, show how they are interrelated, and begin to identify what theory will support such activities and make their success predictable.

Each step in the process should be examined in terms of definition, content, and process: what is a nursing diagnosis, what must be included in it, and how does a nurse go about it? Only when the components are understood fully can relationships between the steps be understood and the process used effectively.

USING THE PROCESS TO DIRECT CARE

During extensive experience in teaching the process, the author has found that it is best learned sequentially, with clinical practice designed to accommodate each section. Each nurse requires a permanent case load of clients ·for whom authority and continuity are assured. Classroom work of only two to three hours a week for five weeks enables nurses to understand the process and use it competently. It works in any setting where nurses treat clients and have time and access to determine care needed, give that care, and evaluate the results. Primary nurses, nurse practitioners, and community nurses are the three models discussed in the following pages who can use the process to direct their care.

Diagnosis: The Beginning and Key to the Process

The process begins when a nursing diagnosis is tentatively identified. Usually the nurse sees a behavior pattern that not only signals an unhealthful response but also points up the causative factors. A nursing diagnosis is a client's behavior or state of being that is unhealthful for that individual. What is unhealthful for one client may be healthful for another. The negative emotions in a unique pattern identified by Kubler-Ross in her work with dying patients are healthful.[1] These emotions are part of the grieving work that allows an ultimate acceptance and peace to emerge. The same emotions (denial, anger, depression) even when healthful must be monitored and drained of their bitterness and destruction by supportive, reflective nursing care. If such responses are healthful for the dying, how can they be labeled nursing diagnosis (unhealthful behavior)? This can and must be done because these responses are potentially unhealthful if not resolved and may become unchanging, prolonged, or inappropriate and therefore harmful to that individual. Nurses work in preventive as well as restorative ways and therefore seek to prevent potentially unhealthful behavior in the dying client. For other clients, the same emotions actually may be unhealthful. For instance, "depression related to feelings of worthlessness" in an aged bed-ridden woman clearly is unhealthful for her and should be of primary and immediate concern to her nurse.

What may seem to be unhealthful behavior to the nurse may not be unhealthful at all. The small child whose diagnosis is "fear of injections" is exhibiting healthy self-preservation behavior. In a more complex example, "excessive anger with staff related to perceived inadequate care" again may be a healthy activity. Sometimes nurses address client behavior that is troublesome for them but may not be unhealthful for the client. These are not nursing diagnoses. Such factors as excessive complaints, loudness, or body odor all may be problems for nurses and may be signs of nursing diagnosis, but they are not diagnoses themselves. A nursing diagnosis involves not only an unhealthful client behavior but also a problem for which nursing therapy is needed for resolution of a potential health hazard. That therapy can be hands on, counseling, or teaching, or may be monitoring and enhancing of a particularly weak but important positive behavior. There can be unhealthful behavior and conditions that require the help of health professionals other than nurses. Those are not nursing diagnoses. For instance, some aggression may require legal intervention, while poor nutrition, if critical, may require acute medical care. However, aggression and inadequate nutrition are nursing diagnoses when complete data interpretation demonstrates that nursing intervention will be different from other therapy and will be helpful in alleviating the problem.

Etiology Makes Therapy Specific

Whether a nurse or another professional should intervene is determined not only by the seriousness of the behavior but also by whether the etiology of that behavior can be addressed by nursing therapy. Inadequate nutrition, even if only a mildly unhealthful state, is not a nursing diagnosis if the cause is intestinal obstruction. In that case, intestinal obstruction is the medical diagnosis and inadequate nutrition a sign of that diagnosis. The signs and symptoms of medical diagnoses often are nursing diagnoses also. As long as the cause of the nursing diagnosis can be ameliorated by nursing therapy, the medical symptom can be labeled properly as a nursing diagnosis.

When a client has an identified medical diagnosis and unhealthful responses (nursing diagnoses) accompany it, they can and should be addressed by the nurse. For instance, cancer patients have extraordinary actual and at-risk nursing diagnoses.[2] In fact, cancer therapy always should include the definition and treatment of nursing diagnoses, for their resolution not only increases comfort and well-being but may be lifesaving in a direct sense.[3] Pain, nausea, immobility, depression, fear, and malnutrition all constitute common and predictable unhealthful behavior in cancer patients that can be ameliorated by professional nursing care, and in so doing, can prolong life and well-being. These are nursing diagnoses that nearly always and predictably accompany medical diagnoses (see Table 3-1).

Other nursing diagnoses occur in a more individualized manner, the causes coming from special conditions in the client's life. Financial problems, family interrelationships, job-related concerns, or self-image and expectations singly or together can cause many kinds of unhealthful states. The unhealthful behavior may not have anything at all to do with the presence or absence of a medical diagnosis. Factors such as overdependence, anxiety, headaches, nausea, or diarrhea, all can be common conditions arising from uncommon sources. In other words, obesity can result from overeating or inactivity, sleeplessness from endocrine disorders, anxiety or pain or nausea from food intolerance, anxiety from eating too fast, etc.

So although a group of clients may have a common unhealthful behavior, there may be a multitude of individual causes. To resolve those common problems, the cause in each case must be determined so that therapy will be targeted effectively. Therapy is cause specific. Pain is treated best only when the cause is known. Pain from pressure is treated differently from pain from ischemia or from dilated blood vessels. Nausea is treated differently if the cause is a virus, or overeating, or medication side effects. It is

---

Table 3-1 Nursing Diagnoses for Cancer Patients

Physiological

Pain related to
- pressure of growing tumor
- obstructed lumen
- nerve root involvement
- pathological fractures
- inflammation/infection

Nausea related to
- chemotherapy
- radiation
- possible tumor metabolic byproduct
- decreased digestive process

Malnutrition related to
- nausea and vomiting
- protein loss (nitrogen balance)

Skin breakdown related to
- low protein balance
- edema
- immobility
- extreme weight loss

Table 3-1 continued

- decreased nutritional state
- circulatory impairment

Infection related to
- depressed body defense system
- therapeutic risks
- tissue necrosis

Noncompliance with therapy related to
- lack of understanding
- nonacceptance of diagnosis (denial)
- depression

ADL deficit related to
- mobility defects

Depression
Isolation
Hostility
Despair
Denial: prolonged/unchanging
Anxiety
Change in deteriorating self-image
     related to
Feelings of
- meaninglessness
- uselessness
- hopelessness
- being a burden

Fear related to
- possibility of loss of function of senses
- loss of dignity
- loss of control
- ability to stand it
- loss of an organ/function
- expected pain
- anticipated death

Source: Reprinted from *Diagnosis for Cancer Patients* by Mary O'Neil Mundinger by permission of Masson Publishing Company, © 1978.

clear that an unhealthful response could only be treated hit-or-miss if the diagnosis lacked information about the etiology of the situation. A nursing diagnosis, therefore, is most complete and effective when it has two clauses: unhealthful response and related (causal) factors. Sometimes the best that can be done is to see that the two factors are related and occur together, even when there is no definite causal link. Sometimes, to say "caused by" would be an untrue or libelous statement. Therefore, linking two clauses by "related to" is the most judicious way to state a nursing diagnosis.

Two Clauses for a Nursing Diagnosis

The first clause in a nursing diagnosis always is a statement of a client's unhealthful state or behavior. It also must be changeable. For example, "blindness" is not an appropriate first clause. The unhealthful behavior associated with blindness—frustration, anger, social isolation, or potential for accidents—provides the nursing concern. A third criterion for the first clause is that there must be data available to validate the diagnosis. Too often nurses have jumped to conclusions about client responses without demanding of themselves or their peers enough conclusive information. Often a diagnosis is an inferential statement. Red skin or edema are unhealthful states that take little inference; they are nearly facts in themselves. Usually, though, an unhealthful response involves an interpretation of facts. For instance, a nurse cannot "see" anxiety. The information to diagnose anxiety more often includes a furrowed brow, poor appetite, inability to concentrate, inability to fall asleep, nervous "picking" gestures with hands, restlessness, and a verbalized sense of vague fear.

The first part of a nursing diagnosis, then, has these characteristics:

1. The client is exhibiting a behavior or state of being.
2. The behavior clearly is unhealthful for that individual.
3. The observation or inference is based on available data.
4. The response identified has the possibility of change to a healthier state.

The second clause (or related factors) also has four criteria:

1. Data must be available to show a relationship between the response and the identified cause.
2. The cause must be able to be changed or mitigated.
3. Nursing therapy must be required as at least part of the resolution.
4. Continued or complex intervention must be necessary.

Data to validate a relationship are a requirement so that no quantum leaps of imagination or supposition occur. Since therapy is cause specific, it is imperative that the cause as well as the response be determined specifically. Both cause and response should be changeable or there is little chance that the response ever will change to a more healthful one.

Just as blindness, in its permanence, is an inappropriate first clause, so is it an inappropriate second clause. If a tentative diagnosis were "depression related to blindness," the nurse would need to go further and ask "What is it about blindness that is causing depression?" The answer may be blindness-imposed social isolation, unemployment, or sense of uselessness. Any of these three more definitive reasons can be changed, making possible the progression from depression to more positive emotions and functioning.

The identified cause also should require continued or complex therapy, including a nursing component. What this essentially says about a nursing diagnosis is that we nurses identify it and nurses treat it. The therapy may include referrals or autonomous activities of other professionals (e.g., medication prescription or physiotherapy regimes) but for the statement to be classified as a nursing diagnosis, its resolution must require some nursing care. A client may experience headache and nausea whenever he is exposed to his wife's favorite perfume. If all that is needed is a one-time intervention to dispose of the perfume, this is hardly a nursing diagnosis. At other times, nursing intervention may be the resolution needed but if it is a one-time occurrence, it hardly deserves to be written up. For example, if a client experienced a painful sensation in his arm from an IV and it was relieved by positioning, the nurse probably would be wasting time to write that up as a process recording. However, if a problem potentially can recur, it does justify being written up even if therapy or prevention is simple and short (e.g., palpitations related to excessive coffee, sleeplessness related to many visitors, skin rash related to alantoin derivatives).

Nursing diagnoses are negative physical and emotional responses. The physical ones are voluntary as well as involuntary. Noncompliance with prescribed therapy may be one of the most common nursing diagnoses and usually is a voluntary physical response. The involuntary physical responses are the more visceral ones—pain, nausea, diarrhea, and the common conditions of decubiti, skin disorders, malnutrition, obesity, and impaired circulation. The list is endless. Any physical disorder that can be alleviated by nursing therapy is a nursing diagnosis.

As nursing knowledge and skill increase, so does the list of nursing diagnoses. Often the cause rather than the response determines whether it is a nursing or medical diagnosis. This is true because therapy is cause specific: if pain is caused from dependent swelling, nursing measures can be very effective; if pain is from tumor pressure unrelieved by nursing therapy, then that is a symptom of a medical diagnosis.

Emotional or psychological responses also can be nursing diagnoses, and again, the cause makes the difference in whether it is nursing or medical. Pathological causes, whether behavioral or physical, are more likely determinants of medical therapy and are considered medical diagnoses.

The same term can be used in the first clause in some instances, and in the second clause in others. This can be confusing, but it is helpful to keep in mind two questions: "What am I hoping to change in my client's behavior?" and "What am I going to pursue with my treatment?"

One example might involve (a) obesity related to overeating and inactivity and (b) potential emboli related to obesity. In this instance, the overeating and inactivity would need to be addressed in order to resolve the obesity, which ultimately reduces emboli potential. A second example could involve (a) immobility related to depression and (b) circulatory impairment related to immobility. Immobility is the unhealthful behavior in the first example, and the cause in the second example. How the diagnosis is written and acted upon depends on what is hoped for in client status. In other words, if depression is the reason for immobility, the nurse somehow must change or solve the depression in order to increase mobility. In the other example, circulatory impairment is the unhealthful state to be changed, and therapy will be aimed directly at immobility, either through passive therapy (range of motion, ambulation, etc.) or through assistive devices and counseling.

Depression, too, can be the cause or the response in a nursing diagnosis. Where it goes in the equation depends on how the nurse views what should be changed in client behavior and what will be addressed as a causal mechanism. Sometimes one has to be resolved before the other. For instance, the diagnosis "depression related to feelings of uselessness" would have to be known and uselessness addressed before "noncompliance related to depression" could be resolved. The desired result may be compliance, but in order to achieve it, the nurse must resolve the feeling of uselessness in order to resolve depression. It becomes a three-step instead of a two-step process. Getting to the cause of the cause is the first step in success.

THREE LEVELS OF NURSING DIAGNOSIS

Nursing diagnosis can involve actual, possible, or potential situations. The differences among the three have been developed using Marlene Mayers' framework:[4]

1. An actual nursing diagnosis:
   a. is occurring now
   b. has data to validate both the response and the cause
   c. is written so that treatment can be given to reverse the response

Example:
"Noncompliance with therapy related to lack of knowledge"
2. A possible nursing diagnosis:
   a. may be occurring now
   b. does not yet have enough data either to validate the response or the cause; in fact, since the presence of the response is questionable, the cause almost surely will be unknown, so, there may be only one clause
   c. is written to lead all care-givers to investigate the possible presence of the response and possible causes

Example:
"possible noncompliance"
3. A potential nursing diagnosis:
   a. is not occurring now
   b. is at risk because of client history, disease process, or based on other similar situations; data should be complete as to the absence of conditions and the presence of predisposing conditions
   c. is written so that all necessary preventive care can be justified and given

Example:
"potential noncompliance with therapy related to denial of disease"

Actual Nursing Diagnoses

Actual nursing diagnoses are the most common in practice. Not every client exhibits them, and they are not always demonstrated clearly by those who do. Sometimes even when glaringly present, their presence may not be acknowledged by the client. Examples are responses that are overly dependent, or due to poor self-image or to denial. All of these are inherently difficult for self-acknowledgment. Because nursing therapy almost always requires client participation, this might seem to be a difficult barrier, but in practice it is not, for client participation revolves around consensus on goals, not problems. The goals for actual nursing diagnoses involve measurable behavior showing an improvement from the problematical state. The evaluation of therapeutic action is aimed at whether or not the initial unhealthful response has changed to a healthier one.

Potential Nursing Diagnoses

Potential nursing diagnoses can be diagnosed (or imagined) for everyone. All individuals are at risk for unhealthy occurrences based on their habits, life style, and environment. Anyone who actually is ill or hospitalized is at risk for a whole list of predictable unhealthy occurrences: infection, anemia, respiratory dysfunction, emboli, malnutrition, anxiety, depression, etc. With this sinister group of potential diagnoses lurking in every corner, how can decisions be made about labeling and acting on them for a client? There is no helpful, easy answer.

The ultimate decision to identify and act on potential diagnoses depends on the nurse's judgment of just how much the client is at risk for developing that condition. Many of the factors that go into the decision are based on that client's past and current health. If the individual is old, weak, debilitated, or already ill, the person is far more at risk for almost any other unhealthful response than is someone with health and strength. The client's past ways of responding to illness or stress also are indicators of how the person will handle current problems. There also are less individualized determinants of risk based on known side effects of disease or environmental conditions. Surgery may be a precondition for pneumonia and infection; bedridden clients are more at risk for emboli and circulatory deficits; diabetes poses risks for many kinds of health problems. Any client who is predictably at risk because of personal health status and history or because of common results of a specific disease or condition should have potential diagnoses listed and preventive action taken.

A key difference in potential nursing diagnosis is that many medical diagnostic labels are legitimate as potential occurrences. Part of the definition of a nursing diagnosis is that nursing therapy resolves it. To treat a potential nursing diagnosis, preventive (not curative) actions are required. Whereas nurses do not treat clients' existing pathology, they do treat those at risk for pathology. Therefore, we do not treat strokes or heart attacks but do treat potential strokes and potential heart attacks, potential emboli, potential infection, and potential self-harm.

Preventive therapy is well within the scope of nursing knowledge and skill. Analyses of medical and nursing education and objectives show clearly that nurses are educated to detect health risks in life style and physical findings and are competent in providing health promotion and disease prevention therapy. Potential diagnoses identifying pathology as the avoidable problem are valid for nursing.

Possible Nursing Diagnosis

Possible nursing diagnosis is a call for watchfulness. Is the suspected response really taking place? A diagnosis may have a validated unhealthful response but the cause is not certain, e.g., noncompliance with therapy related to possible denial or possible lack of knowledge. Nursing intervention would differ markedly for either cause, so this kind of diagnosis is written so that complete and accurate data are obtained to rule out one or both causes.

Medical diagnoses tend to stay the same until they are cured. Not so nursing diagnoses; they come and go and flow into each other even while therapy is working. Kubler-Ross was an early observer of the way responses change, backtrack, go forward again, and detour constantly. This makes evaluation of a lasting outcome difficult.

Physical responses are almost as contrary and unpredictable as are emotional ones. Pain sometimes will go away, even if temporarily, in the absence of therapy or in the midst of the wrong therapy; nausea ebbs and builds under similar conditions. This frustration in working with actual diagnoses is widespread, and the goals and evaluations must be carried out in ways that demonstrate a change in condition or priority.

Success with potential diagnoses has its own set of problems. Success here depends on maintaining the status quo and on preventing interferences from arising. Success means that the feared conditions never occur, and it often is difficult to place a value on absences. Some clients or critical peers may wonder if the risk ever really was there. It is much easier to justify one's actions by a change in the client's condition. If improvement can be developed as one of the goals with potential nursing diagnosis, clients find it more motivating.

Possible nursing diagnoses are those suspected to be actually present but about which data are incomplete. They rarely are written unless the suspected response is so serious that early detection is imperative. Otherwise most of us would use our available time for other activities and would wait to see whether the suspected response became more apparent.

Diagnosis is the key to the nursing process. It directs and gives meaning to all the other steps. Figure 3-1 demonstrates how a carefully determined nursing diagnosis can direct the four other steps that follow.[5]

Figure 3-1 Nursing Diagnosis and Its Role in the Process

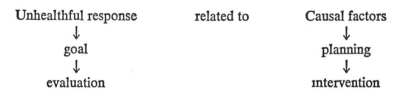

The unhealthful response is the client condition that merits changing. The goal, which flows directly from it, is a client response that is more healthful than the diagnostic one. The evaluation at the end of the process primarily is an analysis of whether the initial unhealthful response has changed to a healthier one; secondarily, the evaluation is to determine whether the goal was reached. (This is discussed in more detail in this chapter's section on evaluation.) Flowing from the second clause of the diagnosis, the causal or related factors, are the planning and implementation steps. Because therapy is cause specific, the planning and the therapy are linked directly to the cause.

Keeping in mind the criteria for formulating nursing diagnosis (four for each clause, listed earlier) and by being aware of the seven deadly sins listed in Table 3-2, the beginning diagnostician can make a measurable impact on solving the client's health problems.

GOALS ARE HEALTHFUL ACHIEVEMENTS

Goals form the next step in the nursing process, the one where clients are much involved. A goal is a measurable, achievable health status and can be the aim of nursing therapy even without a diagnosis. A health goal is a behavior or condition desired by the client. It is a behavior or state that arises from within the individual through expert nursing assessment, motivation, care, new knowledge, new beliefs, new skills and new abilities.

When a diagnosis is identified, the goal follows as an expression of the desired, more healthful response. Two factors tend to enhance the success of goal achievement. The nurse should:

1. Start with an intermediate rather than the final goal. Often the desired final goal seems so far removed from the initial condition that the client will feel overwhelmed in trying to reach it. Instead, the nurse should begin with an improved behavior within easy reach of the client. If independent ambulation is the ultimate goal for a person recovering from a stroke, an intermediate goal might be independent leg raises to 90°, or lifting five-pound ankle weights.
2. Work on client priorities first. Assume this same stroke-incapacitated client had a number of health problems with many possible goals— ambulation, memory, speech, strength—all possible areas for therapy and improvement. If the person can decide the priorities for goal achievement, the client not only will be motivated to follow those choices but will have regained some self-determination and power that is critical for recovery.

Table 3-2 Seven Deadly Sins in Nursing Diagnosis Development

1. Need rather than response
2. Reversal of clauses
3. Unchangeable response or cause
4. Inadvisable legality: libel/liability
5. Not clearly unhealthful
6. Tautology: both clauses identical
7. Nursing rather than client response

Examples and Corrections of Improper Nursing Diagnoses

1. Need
   - fluid replacement related to pyrexia
   - Correct: dehydration related to pyrexia
2. Reversal
   - lack of knowledge related to noncompliance with diabetic diet
   - Correct: noncompliance with diabetic diet related to lack of knowledge
3. Unchangeable
   - inability to speak related to laryngectomy
   - Correct: social isolation related to communication deficit
4. Inadvisable legality
   - red sacrum related to improper positioning
   - Correct: red sacrum related to inadequate circulation
5. Not clearly unhealthful
   - anger related to terminal illness
   - Correct: social isolation and noncompliance with medical regimen related to anger over terminal illness
6. Tautology
   - inability to move bowels related to constipation
   - Correct: constipation related to immobility
7. Nursing
   - suctioning related to thick secretions
   - Correct: choking related to thick tracheal secretions

Source: Adapted with permission from "Developing Nursing Diagnosis," by Mundinger and Jauron, *Nursing Outlook,* © 1975.

When goals are written for factual nursing diagnosis, they flow quite easily. The diagnosis "decubitus related to poor circulation" will have validating data describing the decubitus, in size, location, and condition. The goal, therefore, will describe interim healing—"decubitus will be less than 3″ diameter in one week" or "decubitus will have granulation tissue within ten days."

In developing goals for diagnoses that are inferential (anxiety, e.g.), the nurse must refer to the original data in order to develop a valid goal. "Lessened anxiety" is not appropriate because judgments rather than measurements would be used, and they are too subjective. Goals for anxiety are statements directly related to the behavior that suggested the diagnosis initially. If sleeplessness, poor appetite, weight loss, furrowed brow, and restlessness were the data from which anxiety was inferred, then these form the behavior that must change to more healthful in the goal statements. Goals that are time oriented serve two purposes. First, they start nurses thinking about how long it may take to reach a certain desired condition. Second, they lead nurses back to goal statements on a set schedule for evaluation.

In first working with nursing process development with primary nurses, we found that the time frame stopped somewhere between the implementation of goal-directed activities and the evaluation. Care simply continued, was modified if other factors intervened, or stopped if the client was discharged. Part of the reason for this was that we did not know how long it might take to reach certain stages of achievement, and part was because dates seemed to signal "success" or "failure" when the magic day arrived. The term "assessment dates" was used to avoid confusion with "achievement dates." Whatever the name, dates are important so that goal achievement and actions to reach them can be monitored and evaluated. Determining a goal really means that the nurse has a prognosis for the client. A prognosis is a judgment about a problem's outcome on health.

Some prognoses inevitably are negative with progressive or terminal illness. For instance, ADL (Activities of Daily Living) independence, mobility, and optimal nutrition all are major health areas for which goals may be unattainable for some clients. In the event that deterioration is the only possible future, there still are profitable ways of goal development with a client. Maintaining the status quo as long as possible (the present condition is described as the goal) or the absence of other debilitation (decubiti, pain, sense of worthlessness) can be extremely important for the individual's welfare. Even when promotion or a sense of positive achievement is unrealistic, nursing goals serve the purpose of maintaining a given level of health for as long as possible and avoiding the problems that still are avoidable. Naming those problems ("absence of decubiti will be maintained") tends to mobilize and focus care-givers so that goal achievement is more likely to occur.

There can be goals without nursing diagnoses, and the process can begin with this step. Some persons who have no identifiable unhealthful responses, either real or potential, still have goals for healthful behavior not yet attained. Those who want greater physical endurance or fitness, or an optimal level of low frustration or low anxiety, or to prepare for an extraordinary effort either physical (a marathon swim) or psychological (examinations) are examples of healthy persons with desires for optimal behavior, even in the absence of unhealthful responses. There is, for the purists, a way of developing this kind of optimum nursing process using diagnoses. An overall description could be: "potential severe dissatisfaction related to inability to meet self-selected health goals." It also could be written as an actual nursing diagnosis if the client already is experiencing the dissatisfaction (or depression or frustration).

The desirable health goals in the absence of specific nursing diagnoses are not always self-selected; sometimes it is the nurse who identifies them in the process of obtaining a complete history and evaluating the results of a physical exam. Clients may think that certain valued activities in the past no longer may be possible, or that certain holes in the fabric of their lives are to be expected even if not desired. This is particularly true for the individual who has experienced illness or incapacitation in some form (perhaps financial) that put an end to certain behavior or regimens. Physical exercise is a common example. Once the person has emerged from such a period of disablement, there may be compromised ideas about what is possible for the individual. Young people, who firmly believe they never will grow old or weak, are less prone to this problem. Adults who have not learned to grow and adapt to changing metabolism, muscle tone, and endurance are far more at risk for nonmaximization of health status. Developing new goals or new ways to meet them often are the direct result of identification and therapy from a nurse. The best part about a goal is that it signals accomplishment, which is satisfying to client and nurse.

DATA VALIDATE DIAGNOSIS AND GOAL

Data play a twofold role in the nursing process—they suggest the presence of nursing diagnoses, and they are the proof that diagnoses and goals are valid. Many kinds of data are available in every client encounter. Only part of the information has any place in the nursing process. Some data are keys to diagnosis identification, others are peripheral and not necessary.

For a diagnosis of pain, the client alone can validate the problem. In the absence of client report of pain, all other indicators are inferential at best. Even in the absence of other indicators, a client's report of pain *is* pain.

Data needed for other diagnoses may not be as clear. Noncompliance can be diagnosed by observation, pill count, or presence of effects usually resulting from noncompliance, but none of these is foolproof and the less clear the noncompliance, the more data are needed. Any diagnostician (nursing, medical, legal, etc.) must have available data to validate the therapy prescribed. Much of nursing diagnostic work has been through intuition, which really means the nurse has analyzed a syndrome of signs and symptoms mentally without differentiating one from another. This intuitive element must be seen more scientifically as signs, symptoms, and nurses' uniquely professional judgment to add meaning to the data.

Although the information available to all health care professionals is essentially the same, what is done with it differs and is determined by each professional separately. In each case, data are essential to a valid diagnosis and legitimate therapy.

PLANNING: CAUSE-SPECIFIC THERAPY

Planning is the step aimed at the second clause of the nursing diagnosis —the etiology of the unhealthful response. It takes place concurrently with goal setting or just afterward. The plans are nursing activities, referrals, and coordinating efforts that specifically undo, or moderate the influence of, the cause of the problem. If the diagnosis is correct, and identifies the real cause of the problem, then attempts to change the influence of those causal factors will change the response to a more favorable one. A diagnosis for a person with a chronic disease might be "extreme frustration related to excessively rigid self-care." If this is a valid diagnosis, planning to make a more flexible and less burdensome self-care regimen is the appropriate therapy.

If this is accomplished, the extreme frustration will lessen. Most nurses instinctively want to address the unhealthful response with their therapy, but this is difficult to do. Therapy always is cause specific; it would be unusual indeed to successfully change extreme frustration unless the nurse knew why it was occurring. If success is not achieved, the therapy may not be at fault, but the diagnosis may be incorrect.

In one example, if a measurably different and more flexible self-care routine were adopted and the frustration continued, some other factor probably was causing the frustration. Effective planning depends on identification of the true factors causing the problem.

Planning is a combination of nursing therapy, referrals, and coordinating efforts. Referrals are self-explanatory: asking other professionals to participate in alleviating a client's condition by giving them the data that suggest the need for their independent services. Nursing therapy is the service provided most expertly by nurses through knowledge and skill that is peculiar to their profession. Coordinating efforts are those between professionals, including exchanges of data and progress, and among family, client, and care-givers.

Plans are best when written. Continuity, clarity, retrieval, and monitoring all are enhanced when plans are available to everyone to read and review. The nursing orders (any authoritative plan is an order) include who will carry out an action, when, and how. The authority in a referral is an interesting question. Most professionals welcome the request of another for assistance in the care of a client. Sometimes referrals are inappropriate and may be refused. In those cases, the nurse and the other professional need to reevaluate the data and see what is needed. Nurses are more likely to get inappropriate referrals than to give them. When a client is noncompliant, a physician may ask a nurse to teach the person the expected self-care. Usually the problem is not lack of knowledge but factors such as lack of resources or conflicting or extremely uncomfortable therapies that pose more problems than the health problem being treated. In such instances, no amount of teaching would increase compliance. Rather, the most effective nursing time would be that spent with the physician to devise a regimen more compatible with the client's abilities and motivations.

Coordinating efforts assure that conflicts or overwhelming therapies will not occur and that the client's questions and responses are responded to and observed regularly. The primary therapist always is accountable for the coordinating effort. Clients sometimes have two separate concerns being treated and coordinated, and the diagnostician in each case is accountable for planning and coordinating the therapies to resolve that specific problem. For instance, a person suffering from a myocardial infarction will have a medical plan directed by a physician. The client also may be experiencing "anxiety related to possible marital and occupational disablement" and this diagnosis will be directed by the nurse.

Counseling on exercise, stress, and diet will be key elements of nursing therapy. Reducing weight or giving up smoking may be appropriate goals. The nursing plans are made and implemented as soon as the client expresses a desire to begin. This may be early or late in the medical therapy and depends on individual readiness. At the same time, the nurse may be carrying out part of the medical plan as well as coordinating the various efforts so that the client is not overwhelmed with separate activities for many medical and nursing goals.

Planning or nursing orders have the most chance of success if the client is included in formulating the required activities—the client's own and the nurse's. This step and goal setting are the ones that should be developed with a high degree of client participation. Unlike medicine, which can provide services passively (surgery, chemotherapy, radiation), nursing requires self-help measures and client motivation in order to succeed. Nursing at its best is making optimal health possible for individuals. Health is a continuum, not an end point, and therefore requires transfer of learning belief and skills from the nurse to the client for the latter's own continuing health maintenance and promotion. In order to begin this transfer, there must be consensus on what the goal is and how to get there.

NURSING THERAPY: AUTONOMY AND INTERDEPENDENCE

Implementation is actually giving care, carrying out the referrals, and coordinating efforts. It also includes continuous analysis of new data and new responses as the care is provided. This is the one step in the process that is not new to nursing but is one that takes on new and autonomous meaning in this context.

When care becomes goal directed, it takes on more urgency and meaning than when it simply is a task process arising from medical, institutional, or routine nursing direction. The ideas of nursing autonomy and professionalism as defined by diagnoses and goals are gaining wide acceptance. Health problems identified and solved uniquely by nurses put a stamp of legitimacy on nursing as a profession. The question often remains, however, about the exact content of nursing therapy. The diagnosis and goals may be peculiar to nursing, but are the actions? Is there really a set of therapeutic activities that belongs only to nurses?

Health teaching is an example. Nurses follow common educative principles in teaching new knowledge, beliefs, and skills. To do so, however, we also need to know the specific hazards, risks, and disabilities in the health disease spectrum that pose risks for learning. Few other professionals have knowledge as educators and as detectors and participant-therapists of disease.

Counseling in its generic sense is the purview of other professionals, too: ministers, lawyers, psychologists. What makes counseling a professional characteristic of nursing is that the outcomes (higher motivation for health achievement, greater understanding of various health behavior alternatives) are achieved best by nurses because of their knowledge of health and disease and because of their communication and motivational skills. Physical assessment and history taking in nursing are unique because the focus is health. Where abnormal situations are identified, those that are pathological are referred to a physician and those that can be reversed through nursing care and self-help are addressed independently. Findings that are normal but suboptimum can be made better through client-nurse interactions. This maximum health status can be achieved using nursing knowledge and skill about what health levels are possible and what activities can help reach the desired levels of functioning. Physical assessment and history taking are useful for nursing after primary contact. The same kind of physical and psychological information gathering and assessment goes on to determine progress toward goals and new strategies to reach them.

Persons who do not need physical care may need emotional and psychological care instead. Unhealthful responses, or the absence of some healthful responses, often can be the primary reason for nursing care. Nurses can best identify and treat these responses.

Teaching and counseling for resolution and self-care of disease or pathology are unique elements of professional nursing. Pathology resolution is the scope of medicine; resolution of responses to pathology is nursing. Teaching and counseling are autonomous nursing activities, based on diagnoses that show the cause to be lack of knowledge, belief, or skill for needed self-care. This is probably the finest example of the autonomy and interdependence of nursing and medicine. Each has its separate diagnosis and therapy and each relies on the other's success for full achievement. The client, by receiving appropriate care for problems and deficits, eventually is able to assume self-care for continued and improved health.

Nursing therapy, then, is professional because the knowledge base is unique: pathophysiology, psychology, bodily care, teaching, and counseling. Few other professionals have such repertoires of interdependent knowledge. Nursing is one of the only professions using primary physical and emotional data and intellectual and hands-on skills to identify and resolve unhealthful responses. Physicians have neither a health promotion priority nor nurturing or teaching skills. Health educators primarily are educators who use secondary, referred data for specific problems. Social workers diagnose and treat social dysfunction that can cause unhealthful responses. Physician's assistants obtain primary data but can provide only secondary, medically directed treatment. Only nurses have the full scope for identification and care to resolve health problems. The combination of knowledge and skill is unique. The constant interpretation of responses, close bodily care, and nurturing that allows those judgments is nursing therapy. Helping someone be the healthiest being the individual can be is the professional outcome.

EVALUATION: DID THE DIAGNOSIS CHANGE?

Evaluation has been the fuzziest step in the nursing process because no one was sure who the evaluator was, what was being evaluated, or what should be done with such an analysis. In the context of the nursing process, all these things become clear. The diagnostician is the evaluator. The one who identifies and acts on the problem is the one accountable for the outcome. However, evaluation should be done in a prearranged and objective way so that any interested professional could come up with the same results. It is the change in diagnosis that is being evaluated. The change is toward more healthful behavior if the therapy was helpful.

Evaluation of goal achievement is more peripheral but easier. Goals are the measurable indicators of problem resolution but sometimes are not quite on target and can be achieved without altering the diagnosis. The best way to avoid this is to establish goals that are positive actions. The absence of certain behavior often is open to success through manipulation rather than therapy and may not have any effect at all on the diagnosis. For example, a goal of "absence of crying" for a child displaying a diagnosis of fear or sadness can be accomplished with power sanctions and still leave the child fearful or sad. Absence of involuntary responses, such as decubiti, are more legitimate as goals. Another example of goal achievement without diagnosis resolution is:

- dx: client shows anxiety related to impending surgery (data validating anxiety include sleeplessness)
- goal: client sleeps uninterruptedly for six hours at night
- questionable result: client is given two sleeping pills at bedtime and sleeps six hours but still is anxious (data include restlessness, sweating, and poor appetite)

If goals are well written and complete, evaluation of that achievement probably is sufficient. However, the ultimate success in evaluation is to demonstrate a healthful change in the initial unhealthful response. Evaluations are done on the assessment date. This often is an interim look at progress, but it may be a final assessment, either because the goal was met, priorities for action changed (acute illness, new desires of client, etc.), or the client left the professional's sphere of authority, being discharged, moving, etc. The new care-giver, if there is one, should have the data showing progress to that date.

The interpretation of progress or success in the evaluation step is used as data to begin the nursing process cycle anew. Is the unhealthful response still present or have new ones emerged? Is there, indeed, still a nursing diagnosis? If so, what are the validating data, and are any of them new or different to suggest more discrete causes or more legitimate goals? The process begins again with a new or unchanging diagnosis. The evaluation helps rule out certain causes or goals, or helps interpret data as a different diagnosis. What was interpreted as "anxiety" actually might be "overdependence"; "nausea" might not be the diagnosis, but only a symptom of "fear," which is the real one.

Evaluation is a necessary step in finishing or expanding therapy. Successful resolution can allow new or secondary diagnoses to surface and require treatment, or it can signal the end of needed nursing care for the time being (see Figure 3-2). The full cycle of the nursing process revolves around diagnoses and their resolution. This happens in every setting in which nurses are responsible for the health needs of our clients.

NOTES

1. Elisabeth Kubler-Ross, *On Death and Dying* (New York: The MacMillan Co., 1970), p. 40.

2. Mary O'Neil Mundinger, "Nursing Diagnosis for Cancer Patients," *Cancer Nursing,* June 1978, pp. 222-225.

3. G. L. Nicolson, "Cancer Metastasis," *Scientific American* (March 1979): 66.

4. Marlene Mayers, *A Systematic Approach to the Nursing Care Plan* (New York: Appleton Century Croft, 1972), pp. 30-31.

5. Mary Mundinger and Grace Jauron, "Developing a Nursing Diagnosis," *Nursing Outlook,* February 1975, pp. 96-97.

Figure 3-2 Nursing Process Audit

Primary Nurse _____ Client _____ Room Number _____

Instructions for completing the audit form:

1. Compare the nursing process criteria listed below with the nursing care plan and related nursing information on the client's chart.
2. Check: a. the "yes" column if the nursing process information completely corresponds with the criteria.
   b. the "no" column if the information does not correspond with the criteria.
   c. the "incomplete" column if the information corresponds only partially with the criteria.
   d. the "does not apply" column if the criteria do not apply to this situation, i.e.: if the client has no possible diagnoses, the data question in number 2 would not apply.
3. If the criteria are not met (checked "no") or are met incompletely (checked "incomplete"), specify the omission or error in the adjacent "comments" column.
4. If a care plan consists of multiple diagnoses, each diagnosis and related information must conform completely to each of the nursing process criteria listed below to be rated in the "yes" column. If one part of the multifaceted plan does not conform to a particular criterion, that criterion must be rated "incomplete." The part of the plan responsible for the deficiency should then be identified under "comments."

	Yes	No	Incomplete	Does not Apply	Comments
Nursing Data:					
1.					Are there data to directly support each actual or potential nursing diagnosis? _____
2.					Do the data correspond with, or precede, the date on which the nursing diagnosis was written? _____
3.					Do the data include facts, not just inferences? _____
4.					Are there insufficient data to validate each possible nursing diagnosis? _____
Total					

Figure 3-2 continued

Yes	No	Incom-plete	Does not Apply	Nursing Diagnosis:	Comments
				1. Is change to a more healthful response possible through nursing intervention?	
				2. Is the unhealthful response clearly stated in the first part of the diagnosis?	
				3. Is the related factor clearly stated in the second part of the diagnosis?	
				4. Is the diagnosis properly worded (using the phrase "related to") and free from libel?	
				Are all major unhealthful responses documented in the data found in the nursing care plan?	
				Total	

Chapter 4

Primary Nursing: Making It Happen in a Traditional Setting

Primary nursing provides the components and framework for professional practice. All the concepts that nurses have bandied about—accountability, continuity, collaboration, autonomy—all really take place in this system. Primary nursing is similar to any truly professional model. Each nurse has a permanent case load and is accountable for identifying and resolving health problems for those clients. This chapter turns more personal, being based to a considerable degree on the author's own experiences in developing the primary nursing system.

The nursing needs of acutely ill clients are present 24 hours a day, seven days a week. Peoples' needs for other professional services are not as continuous, and therefore one professional can assume total contact and responsibility for that care. For instance, neither the legal nor educational needs of any client require 24-hour service. Medical needs are more unpredictable in that they can require care at any time, but again, it is a rare occurrence for a physician to be needed in direct attendance for 24 hours a day. Not so with acute care nursing. This poses one of the biggest problems in developing a professional model for nurses. How can one professional nurse assume the continuity and accountability aspects of care when less than one-quarter of the 24-hour, seven day nursing hours can be provided by one full-time nurse? Another problem is the nurses themselves. Most do not consider themselves careerists. Most continue to look at nursing as a vocation, a job.

Nursing has not recruited for the committed, risk-taking individual, and just as well, because there were few nursing jobs satisfying to such a person. Now, though, the profession is beginning to do both: recruit potential professionals and develop work models that use thinking, creative, autonomous nurses.

SINGLE ACCOUNTABILITY AND SHARED CARE

Primary nursing is most successful when one nurse has the acknowledged accountability for an identified group of clients. Just as each hospitalized client has his or her physician, so does the individual have "his nurse" or "her nurse." That person, the primary nurse, determines with the client the goals to be reached and the nursing care to be provided. The primary nurse also coordinates the medically directed regimen for the team of nursing personnel coming in contact with each client belonging to that primary nurse. It is apparent that more than the primary nurse must be the provider when 24-hour care is needed. However, only the primary nurse has the accountability to the client for identifying health problems, setting goals, planning, and evaluating the care. The primary nurse, and the other personnel, give the care when they are present or on duty. If the client's wishes or condition change when the primary nurse is absent, the nurse responsible for the individual at that time modifies the plan and communicates with the primary nurse when it is appropriate.

This dual aspect—one primary nurse who plans the care, and the joint responsibility with all other care-givers—is the key to accountable practice.

When primary nursing is introduced, both primary nurses and their associates (R.N.s with responsibility on other shifts for giving care to that patient) are edgy about the change in function that the new element implies. Inherent in this conflict is the idea, "I am a professional nurse and so is my associate. Why is it legitimate for one of us to plan with such authority over the other?" Two factors can make such a decision valid:

1. The total number of clients is divided equitably among all the potential primary nurses. In this way, each client has a primary nurse. Some of the nurses always will be on duty, and all of them always care for their primary clients as well as some of those of the absent primary nurses. In this way, every nurse is a primary nurse and associate, accountable for planning for some clients and for giving care to to both groups.
2. Nurses who will function in the primary role must have specific training for these responsibilities, including use of the nursing process, leadership skills, and knowledge about change.

The nursing process education can be completed easily in a few hours. The nursing diagnosis development being carried out nationally will provide a comprehensive set of labels for client problems that nurses treat, along with the identifying characteristics and data needed. The goals that signal specific problem resolution are not being developed centrally, nor are the plans to achieve the goals. These must be developed by the primary nurses who are thinking, practicing, and documenting along the lines of the nursing process. This way of thinking and going about work is not new. Many experienced nurses have said to me, "That's the old way, that's what we did in nursing school and it's what we did before team." What they mean is there was a time when nurses were assigned to certain clients and gave all the nursing care to those persons. There was no medication nurse, no treatment nurse, no team leader.

What was not happening then, though, is an important distinction. Although each nurse may have had a specific group of clients for all nursing care, this occurred shift by shift; 24-hour accountability was not part of the package. It might be questioned whether 24-hour planning accountability is appropriate, since those needing that intensive care almost certainly will experience rapid and frequent changes in condition and abilities that would require a change in the nursing plan of care. This argument holds that those in attendance should have the accountability for planning or changing the care.

There are problems in that system. First, if care is on an hour-by-hour basis, no plans can be made. Second, if care should be planned and given as a means of goal achievement, changing and undirected care may or may not end up in reaching the intended goal. Without a planned, continuous, predictable course of action, nurses never will know which actions are useful in reaching any given goal. Yet that is mandatory if nursing is to reach the stage of maturity where its practitioners can offer, with reasonable certainty, a prognosis for their clients based on a given therapy. Without this, nursing remains a process-oriented activity, offering day-by-day responses, with no accountability for success.

To assure clients continuous predictable care that has a direct relationship to health achievement (or nonachievement), all care-givers must perform the same activities in the same way. This happens best when one nurse has 24-hour accountability for planning and directing care. Some changes may be necessary, but more often these will be in the medical rather than in the nursing regimen. When the nursing care plan must be modified, there is a far clearer picture of what works (or does not work) if an overall goal is in mind and if the degree of care change is documented in the plan and in the progress record. These actions produce the best result if only one nurse is accountable.

Other than the 24-hour accountability for planning, liaison with other care-givers, and goal setting, primary nursing's other main difference from the older case method is in identifying and resolving health problems autonomously. Goals can be developed and met without identifying problems to be solved. Obviously that kind of system is not nearly as responsive to client needs because goal setting in isolation sounds optional. Only if the nurse is motivated to talk goal setting with a client will it take place. In the system, however, where problem definition precedes goal setting, there is a sense of urgency and requirement about setting and reaching goals as a means of resolving a problem. Problem definition can be optional, too, unless nurses develop and use criteria that include nursing diagnosis identification for each client. This is the heart and core of nursing's autonomous service and the real difference from the historical "my patient—my nurse" case method.

Many professional nurses, after experiencing the primary nurse role and using the process described here, have observed that it is different from the case method. Although their own previous practice often had included the responsibility and complete care-giving for the same group of clients every day they worked, there is a difference if the client becomes involved in the care planning process and the nurse independently assumes accountability for health achievements. For those who value these serious and often heavy responsibilities, primary nursing works well. The role rarely is comfortable or successful, however, unless all of the capable and willing R.N.s are primary nurses. A system in which a few write orders for the many will not work. However, nurses will follow each other's plans in order to achieve the continuity required for valid evaluation.

FOUR GROUPS NEEDED FOR SUCCESS

Leadership and principles of change also are requisites for a successful primary nurse. The accountabilities and the activities are so different and yet so subtle from other systems of delivering care that a nurse unaware of the pitfalls will fail utterly, even if commitment and knowledge of excellent nursing care are there. Politics, leadership, and maturity are required. Perhaps the best way to see the successful evolution of full-blown primary nursing is to look at the four groups that make it possible—or impossible.

SUCCESS GROUP 1: CLIENTS

The one group that is absolutely necessary, of course, is the clients, and my experience has been that they much appreciate primary nursing. They also are the best advocates of what primary nursing can do, and more than any other group, can mandate its arrival and survival in an institution.

In the hospital where we first introduced this version of primary nursing there are two wings of patient rooms, the new and the old.[1] The old wing, although renovated and bright and shining, does not have bathrooms in every room; there is a male bathroom and a female bathroom at the midpoint of each hallway. The word is out in our community that the first thing to do if assigned to the old wing is to ask for a transfer. The second thing to do, after arriving in the room, is to call admissions and remind that office that the transfer should be prompt. Room assignments in the hospital have been a musical chairs arrangement for years, with people admitted to the old wing, then transferred to the new. Nurses working in the old wing suffered because clients were eager to leave, and did so after the difficult and time-consuming admission was completed.

Partly because of this morale problem, we instituted primary nursing on an old wing unit. The nurses met and divided the clients among themselves, and after successfully finishing a course on the nursing process, began delivering care in this new way.

Our first identifiable success became apparent when clients began cancelling their transfer requests. It took only a day or two with their primary nurse before they opted for that kind of care instead of for a new room with bath. When clients began choosing to trade off their bathrooms for a primary nurse, we knew we were in business.

The second even that told us that primary nursing was as satisfying to the nurse as to the client occurred when we compared the absentee time and resignations on the three existing primary nursing units with the same figures on the other units and found a significant difference in favor of primary nursing. In fact, over a three-year period, when overall nursing personnel turnover was more than 30 percent, we educated and promoted thirty-four nurses to primary nurse and lost only two, one whose family moved out of state and another who took a leave of absence after childbirth. Other primary nurses who moved or became parents stayed on and traveled as long as an hour each way, passing at least six other hospitals on the way. One nurse moved out of state when his wife had a baby and they bought a house they liked, yet he commuted well over 60 miles a day to stay with primary nursing. Many of our own part-time staff worked less than full-time because of family responsibilities. When we decided that primary nurses could only be full-time nurses, many of our part-timers found their family responsibilities now would allow full-time work. The family responsibilities had not changed, but job satisfaction had.

A third and totally unexpected development also validated client and nurse preference for primary nursing. Our hospital serves a population older than those of most community hospitals. The average age on a

40-bed unit often is over 60. Ours is a stable community and that, plus the higher average age, accounts for many of our admissions' being readmissions. Within a year after instituting primary nursing, clients not only had learned that the old wing meant having a primary nurse, some also had begun to ask for their original primary nurse when they were readmitted. Instead of saying "My doctor is Dr. Wilson and I want the new wing," now they were saying "Dr. Wilson is my doctor and Mrs. Roderiguez is my primary nurse." These primary nurses responded in an equally new way. Instead of complaining and asking for housekeeping assistance, they immediately moved the beds themselves to accommodate "my client."

Clients who have talked about their experiences with primary nursing are quite clear about what they observe and like in the system. One of the more telling comments was from a man who told me that the best thing about primary nursing was the longer shifts the nurses worked. His nurse now worked about eight hours instead of the four-hour shifts to which he was accustomed. On further discussion, I found that the nurse who had helped him bathe and have breakfast in the morning never appeared again after about 10:30, but the medication nurse (second shift) was in and out of his room from 10 a.m. to 2 p.m. Continuity had improved.

Clients tire of repeating the same information and same requests to a successive group of care-givers. They recognize in primary nursing the value of having the one knowledgeable in charge nurse who can communicate for them and be their advocate.

Healing and convalescence often are slow and undramatic; getting sicker can be equally subtle, and the changes may be undetected by transient care-givers. The clients know that their primary nurse is more likely to pick up these changes because of the continuity and the acknowledged accountability, and to be more in tune with them when they report something or question their progress. The "my patient—my nurse" relationship identified by Manthey really happens.[2]

Clients also like being included in the development of their plan of care, and it is this collaboration that assures that the plan will be followed. It is true that a system in which nurses follow each other's plans tends to promote acceptance and implementation as written. However, nothing is a stronger force for implementation and maintenance of a regimen than when the client is a coplanner. The sickness role surely is one of the most powerless ones known to mankind. The medical therapies and their alternatives rarely are explained fully to or understood by clients, making them less challengeable.

The isolation of institutionalization and absence of choices in routines or specific therapies increase the imposed passivity. Add to this the anonymity of hospital gowns and the usual horizontal position in which clients find themselves and powerlessness becomes overwhelming. When these people are given a coplanner role with their nurse who does not disappear after rounds, one of the great satisfactions in care becomes apparent. The serendipity in clients as coplanners is that the planned activities do occur because these individuals always are expecting them to and their motivation for participation is high because they helped to determine them.

Given a choice, clients usually will choose a primary nursing system. Hospitals and, in most urban areas, physicians as well, are vying for clients. Clients can mandate primary nursing by demanding to be hospitalized where that system is working. Physicians usually will recommend hospitalization where they have their largest practice, most influence, and—all things being equal—where the nursing care is best. If clients let it be known that they will go only where primary nursing operates, physicians will tend to get privileges in those places or push primary nursing implementation where they already practice.

Administrators listen to clients, to physicians, and to their budget reports. If primary nursing is an effective marketing device, it will be used. The weak link here, obviously, is that people rarely plan to be hospitalized, which usually occurs after they have chosen and developed confidence in a physician. Even a client who is knowledgeable and who values primary nursing rarely will switch physicians just to receive that kind of nursing care. So the real choice for primary nursing arises only when the personal physician has privileges at both a hospital offering that service and at another hospital. Clients must make known to their hospital board members and administrators the real value of instituting primary nursing and opening admitting privileges to M.D.s who then will send their clients there when hospitalization is required. Consumer power can force hospital changes, and consumers who know primary nursing will opt for it almost every time. Nurses need to advise consumers so they can act as effective advocates of primary nursing.

SUCCESS GROUP 2: NURSES

The second group required for primary nursing are the nurses themselves. The group discussed here includes both nursing leaders and practitioners.

Awareness and changes in nursing leadership must come before those in practitioners. The difference in outlook can be threatening for nursing administrators if they do not first see the new picture, because primary nursing means individual accountability without the hierarchical direction inherent in most nursing services. A different problem arises when the leadership understands fully how the new system can work and the practitioners do not or cannot. For us, this happened because the primary nursing system was being developed as it was implemented. Sylvia Carlson had introduced it successfully and creatively at Long Island Jewish Hospital in New York. She used Manthey's concept and built a strong and unique framework analogous to the medical system. She gave a seminar for our nursing staff and in four hours had even the most conservative nurses thinking they had no other choice than primary nursing.

We used much of her experience and research in developing a system that would work for us. Our contributions were the 24-hour accountability and a definite nursing process of six steps (discussed in chapter 3). Our enthusiasm over the system outpaced what actually was occurring. We would get requests from colleagues in other areas to inspect our primary nursing operation. We would have liked to open a door in our heads and show them the vision of what should be and will be, but instead, we did what was expected and took them to see a primary nurse in action. All too often, they were the same primary nurses, overworked as models for us as well as practitioners for their clients.

As with all pioneers, we kept making changes as we went along, which made it difficult for those who were trying to master this new model of practice. Differences that were subtle but important to those of us leading the effort seemed unnecessary or unrealistic to those trying to implement them. For instance, we believed that a primary nurse should have 24-hour accountability for planning and yet that the nurse in attendance should modify the plan if needed. We believed that only R.N.s could function as primary nurses and yet a licensed practical nurse might be the nurse in charge of giving the prescribed care to a group of clients on a given day.

The L.P.N./L.V.N. or the part-time R.N. are accountable in the primary nurse's absence or time off duty for giving care and modifying plans if required (e.g., ambulation directed in a certain way might be changed or deleted if the client experienced an episode of chest pain or weakness). Often they would voice the frustration that they were doing the same things as the primary nurse. Only when these same R.N. s became full-time and put the nursing process into action could they see and experience the difference. In many ways, all education works this way. Who knows better how philosophy changes life than one who has studied it? Usually those who argue for equal footing (or prestige or acknowledgment) are those who measure the process's sameness ("I do the same thing") rather than outcome ("I accomplish the same thing"). Those who argue against further education (especially opponents of a baccalaureate degree requirement for nurses) base it on the comparison of activities and skill competence (again in process, not outcome). What education will do is to show why and for what purpose activities are carried out. Education gives a nurse a way of looking at those activities in terms of what they can improve in a client's health status. As in so many endeavors, the difference cannot be seen by the uninitiated.

We believed that all primary nurses should be R.N. s. The position is endowed with a high degree of autonomy, accountability, and individual decision making. It seemed to us that clients deserved to have only the most highly qualified practitioner in charge of the task of identifying and resolving individual health problems.

Along the same lines, we believed that only the baccalaureate trained nurse should have these responsibilities. When the primary nurse project began, only one practicing nurse in 200 at our institution had a B.S. degree. Three years later, 34 R.N. s were part-way through an upper division B.S.N. program and we had hired a number of B.S.N. degree nurses. We knew we were on shaky ground saying that baccalaureate practice somehow was different or better because more sophisticated groups of nurses than ours were having trouble nationally demonstrating a clear, clinical difference. We based our decision on several factors:

- National proposals recommend professional licensure for B.S.N. only, and primary nursing definitely is the professional model.
- Our definition of nursing diagnosis included emotional, psychological, and physical unhealthful responses and we felt that nurses needed theoretical courses in chemistry, pathophysiology, sociology, psychology, and group process to even begin to fulfill these responsibilities. Generic undergraduate courses in these areas (not "just for nurses") rarely are offered in diploma or A.D. (Associate Degree) programs. We wanted our baseline to be minimum professional competency.

Many existing primary nursing systems utilize L.P.N./L.V.N.s as primary nurses. In such a system, nurses of different educational levels are assigned to clients on the basis of the complexity of those individuals' medical condition. For instance, the L.P.N./L.V.N. might be primary nurse to a client with an appendectomy whereas a baccalaureate R.N. would be assigned to one undergoing open heart surgery. In a system where primary nursing accountability is for planning and delivering only dependent care to clients, this makes sense. However, we saw primary nursing as a model that could demonstrate the autonomous scope and outcome of professional nursing, which might or might not be related to the medical pathology. For example, the appendectomy client may experience severe anxiety related to fear of anesthesia, noncompliance with restrictive activities related to threat to self-image, or pain and nausea related to paralytic ileus. These responses require complex and sophisticated nursing care and counseling; the L.P.N./L.V.N. may not even detect the problems, much less have the repertoire of skills to resolve them effectively. The open heart surgical client, on the other hand, may be accepting and knowledgeable of hospital care and need only the constant, predictable, skillful physical care and monitoring that L.P.N./L.V.N.s can learn and perform well. It is a paradox that a client must have a primary nurse in order to determine whether one is needed. Only when a qualified and able primary nurse has been in attendance, looking at the data (verbal, behavioral, laboratory, x-ray, etc.) can the real or potential problems (diagnoses) that signal the need for intervention by a primary nurse be identified.

Medical condition has been the pivot for defining health care for so long that it is difficult to look at individual health as the category, with the illness state as only one element to determine care. Most nurses are at ease in defining their care in terms of medical conditions. Therapies to resolve medical problems are more predictable because physicians for years have used the problem-solving process with appropriate documentation. The body of knowledge has grown so systematically and so well that predictions of successful regimens and prognosis for resolution are well known. Concurrently, the complementary nursing activities also have been defined, but have been documented and communicated poorly. During this time nurses often identified and resolved unhealthful responses, useful and creative approaches were devised, and people learned how to improve their health. Primary nursing holds (among other things) that each client has a nurse accountable for identifying and resolving health problems, both real and potential. Primary nursing assures clients that this area of their health care will be addressed. The documentation of such care assures widespread communication with other nurses about what signs and symptoms signal what problems, and what therapies work to resolve them. When nurses can accept this subtle, important area as their own, primary nursing can be the framework to put it all together.

In my experience, nurses learn the nursing process system easily. Accountability for practice oriented to health outcome is assumed enthusiastically and with the same selfless commitment with which nurses have practiced under medical direction. Many of the new B.S.N. graduates come looking for this kind of system; most of the older, conservative nurses, after initial hesitation, learned to value and accept it fully as well. Nurses always have had brains, but they have not always used them for independent thinking; in primary nursing, this liberating activity takes place. If primary nursing could be developed with clients and nurses in a vacuum, it easily would become the most satisfying and prevalent form of nursing care. Unfortunately, it does not happen that way, and administrators and physicians also have goals to meet in their searches for excellence in client care. Some of these goals are in conflict with the development of primary nursing.

SUCCESS GROUP 3: ADMINISTRATORS

The eternal triangle in institutional care has been nursing, medicine, and administration. Usually two of the three form the majority force for decision making. Because nurses have been employees for so long, with their survival based on being paid a salary by administration, the nursing-administration duo has worked together most often. In recent years, nurses have become more aware of and eager for a fuller professional role and have unionized, usually leaving their nurse leaders straddling the fence between administrative and professional goals. Physicians who have seen fat hospital budgets squeezed thin now are fighting for expenditures that historically always were made in their favor. Hospital administrators who often were physicians, now have Ph.D.s or degrees in management instead, and a peer relationship physicians never foresaw and never wanted has developed. Although nurses, physicians, and administrators all want the best care possible for the clients they serve, the three groups see the components of excellence differently. These differences influence the success of primary nursing.

Administrators see primary nursing as an expensive system that requires intensive education and tends to attract independent nurses, who work as client advocates in demanding that still more changes be made. Administrators sense that these nurses tend to see themselves not as employees but as professionals. The administrators are right on all counts. The changes in nursing outlook and expectation, however, are occurring regardless of primary nursing. Perhaps it is a result of the kinds of people entering nursing, or partly the liberation movements, or changes in the educational system. But it is happening.

The other aspect of the administrative view of primary nursing—expense —initially involved the cost of implementating inservice education. This can be a broad and expensive operation. Our own pioneer effort used two educators almost full time for a year and paid on-duty conference and class time for the forty participants, which averaged thirty to forty hours for each nurse. Staffing dollars did not increase with primary nursing implementation.

The same nursing staff, in number and ratio of R.N. to non-R.N., was used in the system in effect before primary nursing. We began by using primary nursing only on the day shift. The program was so new that we all felt the need to be present together as we worked it out. This presented two major problems: (1) either all the patients had to be divided among the day shift R.N s. (a tremendous case load of ten) or some clients would not have a primary nurse; (2) nurses on other shifts resented what they regarded as one more instance of day shift elitism, and they were resistant to carrying out the nursing plans and documentation devised by the primary nurses. When we were able to implement the system over all three shifts, we found that both problems disappeared.

The second expense, after education, is the higher primary nurses ratio, which is optimal for the system. Again, even without primary nursing, a higher R.N. ratio may be developing everywhere, perhaps as a reflection of the shorter length of hospital stay being mandated. No longer is there a large number of relatively stable convalescent clients, and the existing group on the average will be sicker and require more skilled care. The higher expectations of nurses today also generate pressure for more professional hands at work with clients. In addition, the number of nursing personnel has dropped everywhere as hospitals fight to keep shrinking budgets in the black, and as numbers drop, those departing usually are the nonprofessionals. For all of these reasons, the R.N. ratio has become higher independent of primary nursing. Primary nursing implementation, however, also is a compelling reason to increase the R.N. percent of the nursing staff.

Expectations (and perhaps even requirements) for individual health problem resolution are part of primary nursing. In order to provide this service for every client, there should be a primary nurse: client ratio of no more than 1:5. (The nurse obviously may give care to more than five, but the primary responsibility should be for no more than five.) In this system, most of the contact and care is given by the primary nurse, so the number of helpers needed decreases. No longer do nurses believe that care they supervised can be given as effectively by someone else. Rarely are tasks that simple. Each task becomes part of a plan, part of the data collection, part of the evaluation, part of the rapport building. And primary nurses are finding the value and time-saving aspect of greater clinical contact with their clients.

Because the most qualified nursing personnel have the widest repertoire of skills, the nonprofessionals will be missed least in a cutback because all of their activities can be performed by the professionals. Many of the routine tasks regularly performed by nonprofessionals are scrutinized carefully by the professional who must assume them, and many are discontinued or carried out only after determining who really needs them. It is not necessary to devote the same time as before to provide optimum care.

What all this means is that the R.N. ratio can increase while the total number of care-givers decreases, and the total salary increase may not be proportionate to that of the R.N.s. For every R.N. increase, there may be a 1½ decrease in nurses' aides; for every two R.N. gains, three L.P.N./L.V.N. s may be dropped. Not only is efficiency served by having more highly qualified persons available (a choice is made about what is actually needed and more than one task may be accomplished per contact) but the data gathered and therapy given during routine tasks are of higher quality.

Nurse administrators would do well to plan increased R.N. ratios as part of an attrition program as nonprofessionals leave. The increased cost of higher R.N. ratios can be argued as an investment rather than an expense. Nurse turnover is extremely expensive. Del Bueno computed the cost of recruiting, hiring, and orienting each nurse to be close to $2000.[3] In a primary nursing system, the satisfactions have proved deterrents to absenteeism and resignations.

Primary nursing also is a marketing device for hospitals vying for clients. Primary nursing's value as an investment factor is demonstrated because the system legitimately can increase length of stay (which fills empty beds and adds to revenues) although for the same reasons it should decrease readmissions. The seeming paradox in this is that clients are discharged from hospitals when their medical condition is stable and they no longer require intensive 24-hour care. Rarely are the health maintenance goals included in discharge criteria. For almost every chronic disease—diabetes, heart, liver, renal—the medical crises are over before optimum self-care and preventive activities can be learned and internalized. Only when clients have the knowledge, motivations, and skills to maintain and promote health, can they be expected to go home and stay home.

The rubber band phenomenon is disheartening: patients bounce in and out of hospitals for critical care with no time available for the counseling and mastery of health maintenance that keeps them healthy and out of the institutions. If nursing diagnoses are developed that show potential or at-risk health status for clients, discharges may be deferred and the stay lengthened. For instance, if a newly diagnosed diabetic has been hospitalized and the blood sugar levels stabilized with insulin and diet, that person may be ready medically for discharge. However, chances are that that individual will be readmitted for one of the following reasons: high blood sugar level related to dietary noncompliance or to inappropriate insulin coverage for increased activity levels/illness, ulcers related to poor skin care, lack of knowledge of cardiovascular diabetic problems, visual problems, renal problems, coma, or shock, all related to inadequate compliance with the diabetes and medical regimen.

Client and family counseling, education, and supervision can make the difference in decreasing the number of readmissions for many diabetics. Sometimes, only a day or two longer hospital stay, with a primary nurse aware of the client's individual health needs, can result in a longer period of health and productivity after discharge than would occur without this professional nursing activity. Obviously, with length of stay requirements being mandated regionally, administrators cannot expect to be reimbursed for longer stays based on these preventive kinds of nursing needs until the activities are accepted nationally (and regionally) as part of discharge criteria. Health maintenance activities must be articulated by nurses as part of their PSRO (Professional Standards Review) role. What administrators must know is that primary nurses are best able to identify and act on these nursing diagnoses, and the primary nursing system is the one to employ in providing such care.

If administration can resolve the cost/investment considerations, the change to primary nursing will influence the kind of nursing administration needed and the changes throughout the hospital that also will occur.

ADMINISTRATION CONTINUED: NURSING CARE
COORDINATOR

Nursing administration first must recognize and welcome the individual nurse accountability and client decision making that is part of primary nursing. Historically, client care decisions were made by the head nurse. In my experience, head nurse groups should be the first to participate in their changed role and expectations so that they will be able to yield the decision making that is legitimate for the primary nurse. Head nurses' resistance to change is much less if they have new and expanded responsibilities before being asked to relinquish the old.

In traditional settings, head nurses function as liaison between physician and nursing staff, arbiter of disputes among that staff's members, and decision maker for daily assignments and nursing care activities. Often, this responsibility is assumed by supervisors on other shifts even though different nurses take charge on evenings and nights. In primary nursing, the client assignments are permanent and often decided by the primary nurses. Physician liaison becomes more direct, from primary nurse to physician, and far more client centered and collegial as the two get to know each other well in the care of their clients. The head nurse deprived of these important duties may be resentful of primary nursing and denigrate it if new and more demanding responsibilities are not developed. As head nurses see the need for new and expanded responsibilities they are more likely to relinquish the clinical decision making previously practiced. As the clinical judgments are assumed by the primary nurses, the head nurse title is no longer descriptive of the way practice is organized in that service. The new title chosen by our head nurses was Nursing Care Coordinator (NCC) because it was a better description of the new role and responsibilities. The hierarchy depicted in staff nurse–head nurse–supervisor became artificial, and the supervisor category was abolished except for those serving as hospital-wide assistant administrators on the evening and night shifts. Those previously in nursing supervisor positions filled open NCC positions. Supervision of nursing care was in the hands of the practitioners.

Two of the most important new role responsibilities for NCCs were those of quality control agents and staff developers.

Quality control involves regular observance of the clinical care provided by each primary nurse and the process used in planning that care. The nursing process is a tool for assessing quality as well as for planning care and evaluating problem resolution. Each step in the process can be developed, with criteria, so that each primary nurse knows what is expected in the clinical decision making. For instance, in data gathering, the key factor assessed is thoroughness (client interview, physical evaluation, review of medical admission progress notes and related reports such as laboratory, x-ray, physiotherapy, social service, and family interview, and observations). Timeliness is another criterion (initial client assessment and history within the first 24 hours, or even critical elements within the first hour) and appropriateness (depending on medical, emotional, or age status). The diagnosis category can be assessed in terms of supporting data (both adequate and appropriate) and validation of the problem and the cause (through further testing, observation, or interview). The goal also can be audited (appropriate, reasonable, time limited, discussed with client) as can the plan (thoroughness, appropriateness for goal achievement, reasonableness, well defined).

The NCC's clinical observation of primary nurses' skills and thoroughness is necessary for quality control and staff development. The development is directed by the deficits in the intellectual and physical components of care listed above. The evaluation step in the nursing process should be shared regularly between the primary nurse and the head nurse, for it is an objective measure of clinical and intellectual effectiveness. However, the nurse who uses available data still may not meet with success, and the NCC will not equate effective problem resolution with excellent primary nursing. The two can be independent and unrelated. The NCC must look at process as well as outcome. Did the primary nurse identify and use all available data, thoughtful planning, and skillful care? If so, failure to achieve the goal may have little bearing on the quality of nursing; perhaps what is missing for that nurse is not yet available in the profession's repertoire of predictable successes, or perhaps the client and family cannot or will not provide the data or motivation needed for effective problem resolution.

The NCC also must monitor and assess the quality of other areas of primary nursing excellence. An important area is communication. Because the primary nurse's role is such an autonomous one, nurses who do not value collaboration, suggestions, and modifications are not required to seek them. This limits their client planning and interpretations to only their own ideas, and their clients may not receive the comprehensive care afforded by the experience and insight of a group of nurses. Although the system provides for the autonomous role, autonomy does not mean isolation. Nurses must learn to assume an autonomous role with individual accountability, and to make that a legitimate role by communicating their thoughts with their peers, testing their assumptions, and sharing their failures as well as their successes. This method of operation can and must be promoted by the NCC. "How did you arrive at that diagnosis? With whom have you shared your diagnosis? Has anyone suggested alternative goals? How have your colleagues planned for that in the past?" These kinds of questions guide nurses in moving toward accountable practice.

As in every other endeavor, the nursing care team will function more cohesively and productively if the members have had an opportunity to provide input into the data gathering and planning. Rarely will a group blindly follow a plan devised by an isolated (if brilliant) primary nurse. NCC s can foster this kind of input by counseling the primary nurses and, most effectively, by being role models for this kind of decision making. This can be accomplished by the NCC's meeting with primary nurses to determine criteria for the latter's performance and by sharing the goals of the new NCC role.

In addition to communication within the nursing team or component, communication outside that unit also is important, different, and best fostered by the NCC. Historically, the head nurse handled interdepartmental concerns and communications. Areas involved with clinical work now become the province of the primary nurse, although nonclinical and generic policy ones still are managed most effectively by the NCC. For example, a new policy for preparing clients for a diagnostic test would be communicated best through the NCC. If, however, there were a problem with a client's preparation, the communications should be through the primary nurse. This will not happen if the NCC does not allow it and promote it. The only NCC who resigned during our initial changeover to primary nursing was the one who observed, "I was primary nurse to 40 patients and I loved it. Now it's not so much fun. I'm not a teacher and I don't like the second level rewards of watching someone else do something well. I want to be a primary nurse."

Other hospital department members may not like the advent of primary nursing. It may require their knowing, searching for, and waiting for many primary nurses instead of one easily identified head nurse. After all, the head nurse usually was at the desk and could handle all the problems. An interesting phenomenon in observing institutional relationships is that nursing department firstline personnel's achieving such antonomy suggests something illegitimate to chiefs in other departments. For example, should not a supervisor in the finance department communicate only with other supervisors? The hierarchy change in primary nursing begins to be seen as inappropriate by other department heads and can lead to militancy for the same recognition by firstline workers in other departments. At the same time, we nurses always have seen ourselves on a somewhat peer level with the director of dietary but not with the dietary workers. A whole class struggle rears its ugly head. Fortunately, the NCC can resolve this fairly effectively on grounds of education and professional responsibilities and by communicating the change in primary nursing as encompassing mainly clinical decision making and authority for individual practitioners giving care to clients.

Another big change for the NCC in implementing primary nursing is a new role as staff developer. In a hierarchical nursing department, a centralized education department is efficient and effective. When the changes required by education are mainly technical or procedural, the centralized department makes sense. Orientation, new procedures, and updates of deficits that show up in audit activity are well provided by a central education department. However, when the NCC is involved regularly in a clinical audit of how primary nurses go about their work, the development needs identified are met best by individual counseling, coaching, and role modeling by the NCC.

This is the kind of staff development that flourishes in primary nursing. This is not the formalized teaching plan, class time, and behavioral objectives that are necessary and useful in a horizontal educational endeavor. It is more an in-depth and personal enhancement of individual practice.

Obviously, as in any teaching venture, the teacher gains as much as the learner. Working closely with the primary nurses, complementing (and complimenting) and motivating their practice, can be one of the most rewarding experiences for the NCC. The other executive duties on the unit, including budget, staffing, and ordering of supplies, all begin to take less time as the NCC returns to clinical nursing as role model, staff developer, and clinical observer. Many of the clerical tasks are assigned to those who, it now develops, can do them easily.

Perhaps the head nurse could have been equally involved clinically under a team or functional system. The problem with that, however, is that different nurses perform different activities on a daily basis in team nursing. Much time is given to assigning nurses and getting reports from them, then assigning nurses on the next shift and communicating needed information to them. Individual nurse development is almost impossible if roles change daily and followup takes weeks and if there are no authoritative plans with agreed-on goals toward which to work. Saving the time no longer needed for assignments and reports provides time for staff development. Permanent assignments and a working nursing process provide access and framework for individual primary nursing development. Without the components of time, access, and framework, the head nurse rarely will become involved in clinical activity. Because the primary nurse also has those same three components available, the NCC's role modeling and development are expected and usually welcomed.

Initially, a nurse may be uneasy about the clinical inspection by the NCC and also may be protective of the newly won autonomy and authority. Again, one of the best ways to promote productive clinical encounters between NCC and primary nurse is for them to agree mutually on components of expected practice so that both can speak to measurable, objective findings in the audit process. The NCC may find in the audit that one primary nurse regularly is making inferences regarding a diagnosis based on minimal data and a great deal of guessing. Perhaps what has been skimped on is direct data from the client. Instead of saying "Your diagnostic process is weak, I don't think you're getting enough information from your client," the NCC might say, "We've agreed that a requirement for a diagnosis is verbal and physical assessment data directly from your client. I don't see evidence of physical assessment data in your record. Can we discuss how you are getting all the data you need?"

Changing Staffing, Performance Requirements, and Expectations

There are other duties for the NCC that are present in any system but that change in focus in primary nursing. For instance, assuring that the staff comes to work on time, providing equitable vacation and holiday time, and solving conflicts between nurses and clients or coworkers all continue in the primary nursing system. These scheduling and coordinating requirements become more acceptable to nurses when they are decided on the basis of how they will affect the quality of nursing care given than when the rationale is simply "it is policy to do so." Nursing activity becomes a means to an end rather than an isolated behavior.

Staffing becomes a way of assuring the best possible care for clients instead of honoring requests based on what is good for nurses. Conflict resolution sometimes may require assigning a client to another nurse. There are times when certain nurses and clients cannot build the rapport necessary for effective care. When this occurs, it is entirely appropriate for nurses to switch clients. Primary nurses need to hear that personality conflicts with clients are expected at times and are entirely acceptable. What is not acceptable is to maintain the relationship.

Many questions are raised by staff when permanent assignments are considered. The client conflict is one. More often nurses are concerned about whether one nurse will have the heaviest client load and will need more help than a nurse with a lighter load. Another concern is over who will get the problem client. Still another is how other staff members will be assigned to complement the primary nurses. The NCC is vitally important in answering these questions.

The idea of heavy versus light case loads seemed like a very real possibility when we began primary nursing. What actually happened was enlightening. We learned that heavy almost always meant physical care—clients who needed a great deal of hands-on nursing care. Usually these also were the ones who were most acutely ill and least able to focus on or identify their emotional or learning needs. As clients became less dependent physically, they were more likely to have psychological responses that needed attention from the primary nurse, or were ready for the health maintenance counseling and teaching that follow most sickness. In other words, when physical needs are high, clients' learning needs are less in demand, and vice versa. Even with a very sick person, such as a client with a myocardial infarction, the see-saw of physical and emotional needs can be observed.

Nursing always has weighed the physical aspects of care and seen the teaching/counseling role as secondary. This probably accounts for identification of clients needing primarily physical care as a heavy case load. As nurses worked with a group over a period of time and found nonphysical problem resolution was a necessary component of professional care, they began to identify differences in case loads in terms of physical care/emotional and teaching care rather than heavy/light. Interestingly, nurses can be equally busy and productive with both kinds of care, but the kind of assistant needed will differ markedly.

We found in our project that primary nursing worked best when all care-givers for a group of clients were permanent. This meant that the primary nurse would maintain contact and authority with the same group of clients and with the same group of coworkers for those clients (see Table 4-1 at the end of this chapter). This system provides continuity for clients, less time lost in orienting and communicating information and expectations among care-givers, and a sense of pride and comradeship on the team. All full-time R.N.s were given their permanent case load of primary clients.

The number of primary nursing positions never is filled—there is no ceiling. As more full-time R.N.s are hired or substituted in the staff, the number of clients per nurse is adjusted downward so that the case loads become smaller for each primary nurse. All part-time R.N.s, because their educational and legal limits of practice equal those of full-time R.N.s, can assume the full care-giving and decision-making role for clients during the time they are present in an associate primary nursing position. This means that on any given shift, an R.N. associate primary nurse has accountability equal to that of any primary nurse for giving patient care. What the associate does not have is accountability for planning, goal setting, and evaluating activities, nor the overall accountability for teaching coworkers or serving as primary contact/advocate for a group of clients. These activities are not legitimate for part-time professionals because they lack the time and availability required to make such a system work.

It seemed to us that the L.P.N./L.V.N. should not hold an associate role because neither the educational nor legal boundaries of L.P.N./L.V.N. practice suggested independent decision making or care giving for a group of clients. In team nursing, the head nurse maintains control, direction, and accountability for all care. This allows R.N.s and L.P.N./L.V.N.s to practice interchangeably and similarly. Primary nursing demonstrates the differences inherent in professional versus dependent practice and rules out interchanging R.N.s with L.P.N./L.V.N.s.

Nurse's Aides Still Valuable

Obviously, this system is not satisfying for L.P.N./L.V.N.s. The nursing administrator who recognizes their shrinking effectiveness in the primary nursing system will find it productive to replace those positions with R.N.s. The nurse's aide position, however, remains valuable in the system for repetitive physical tasks that do not always require a professional's hand.

Aides are happy in primary nursing. We thought they would miss their patient assignments and resent being given tasks in nurses' plans of giving care. Instead, they felt an enhancement of their satisfaction in their work for two reasons that they shared readily with us: (1) it was "good to have one boss instead of many," and (2) they felt a bond of belonging and caring from their primary nurse that had been missing before primary nursing. Many of the aides related a growing sense of trust and mutual accomplishment with their nurse, and reported learning more than ever before. The primary nurses were making efforts to build rapport on these new permanent teams, and the personal attention, explanations, and teaching they offered the aides was appropriate in enriching care for clients.

Some of the new activities, however, were not as appropriate, although they too were directed toward building rapport. We noticed that primary nurses were observed making beds and picking up around their units more often than before. They had noticed that most of the assignments given their assistants were physical tasks, while most of the intellectual (soft) work was being done by themselves. Nurses who are making a priority of intellectual work while others are hustling about often become edgy and unsure of the fairness in such a division of labor. The result, as we saw it, was that nurses would share in the routine work to show they were not above it and because they felt guilty doing the diagnosing, planning, and counseling while others were doing the tiring and often dull, yet necessary, chores.

Building new values and feeling comfortable with newly formed standards does not come easily. The NCC and other nursing administrators must be present to reinforce the client care excellence that comes only when those best prepared for a job are the ones doing it. This means nurses do the nursing. As far as nurses' doing the nonnursing as well, the administrator must help them see that the trade-off is that they cannot give professional nursing care when they are involved in less specialized pursuits. Time is finite. For every hour a nurse is involved in nonnursing, a client is deprived of professional care. That trade-off cannot be tolerated, even to improve relationships.

NCCs must articulate clearly to all their staffs the value of everyone's working at the top of their abilities, which is true collaboration and team work. What is valuable is to have each participant aware of the need and value of others and to work in a group way to enhance that collective excellence. Nurses who for too long have seen themselves interchangeable with L.P.N./L.V.N.s and team members often doing the same thing as nurse's aides find it difficult to initiate and be comfortable in the primary nursing role. The NCC can help make that happen. One of the key differences between primary and team nursing is that care-givers are assigned to the primary nurse for a group of clients, while in team, the care-givers are assigned to clients. A more subtle difference is that primary nurses are involved physically every day in assessing their clients and in giving at least some of the care. In team nursing, all care can be given to some clients by other than a professional nurse.

The kind of primary nurse plan that is devised by the NCC encompasses the appropriate use of various levels of care-givers and of a back-up system. This back-up involves carryover from shift to shift and providing optimum care even with staff absences. We have discussed how all clients are divided equitably among all full-time R.N.s on all shifts. When the staff is larger, the number of primary clients can be higher because the nonprimary case load will be low. For instance, on some days there may be four R.N. s and four aides on duty for thirty-six clients. Each R.N. will have nine clients to care for, five of whom will be the primary case load. All nine will receive care from that nurse on that shift, with the assistance of one aide. On nights, however, there may be only two R.N.s and two aides, so that each R.N. will deliver care to eighteen clients with the assistance of one aide. The primary load must be much smaller because the nonprimary care-giving is provided to so many more clients. On nights, then, the primary case load may be two.

Coping with Staff Absences

How are unexpected absences filled in the primary nursing system? Essentially there are isolated miniunits of two to three care-givers per ten to fifteen clients, and one absence can double the workload on any given primary nursing district. Our vision of primary nursing was more vertical than horizontal and could accommodate such absences. Because the care-givers for any group of clients was stable and the same over all three shifts, an absence of any one was made up for on the other shifts. For instance, if the aide on days was ill, more baths and once-a-day care was given on evenings for that group of clients. In team or functional nursing, the deficits had to be made up that same shift; horizontal personnel moves were needed and people had to be floated onto that client unit on that shift. If, however, it is the nurse who is absent, a different kind of shift is made, and a primary nurse from another district becomes professionally accountable for both districts with the assistance of both aides. Again, nonpriority care for both client districts is to be assumed by the following shift. In this instance, all the routine physical care may be accomplished as planned (because the full complement of aides was present) but the professional care planned (counseling, teaching, data collection) may be done on the following shift when the full complement of professionals is present.

In planned absences (vacation, leave-of-absence) we experimented with a number of alternatives:

- We added more ancillary staff and assigned the one remaining primary nurse to assume only the professional responsibilities for both districts. This quickly became overwhelming and unmanageable because as soon as staff learned to differentiate professional and nonprofessional activities and to value the newly developed intellectual professional activities, adding a nonprofessional did little to alleviate the double case load of one primary nurse.

- We assigned the NCC to assume that primary nurse district as role model and clinical refresher. It is easy to discern why this failed: the NCC had solidified the new expectations of that job and they could not be dropped to assume the position of the absent primary nurse. The frustrations were greatest among the best NCC's who had made an effort to develop their new roles fully.

- We thought then that there could be an elite squadron of primary nurses who could float to clients missing their own nurse. This might work, but we never found R.N.s who had the makings of good primary nurses and also were willing to change case loads at random. In fact, one similar project gives the flavor of client commitment in primary nursing: One unit where primary nursing was developing accepted all clients on isolation in the hospital. The nursing care often was lonely and slow moving, with much valuable time spent in repetitive procedures and with little family contact. In our administrative omniscience, we decided that the primary nursing in that district needed relief and we proposed a regular six-month rotation to a more sociable district. The primary nurse there was aghast at our proposal and strongly defended a truly permanent assignment to "my" clients. Needless to say, we learned an important lesson about permanent case loads.

- This same acceptance and commitment was evident in the way primary nurses responded to 'problem patients' being part of their permanent clientele. Previously, everyone took turns with the complainer, the physically repulsive, or the resistant client. Care was given, often perfunctorily and quickly and, with a breath of relief, the undesirable was relinquished to yet another care-giver the next day. The concern nurses had about owning such a client quickly became concern about solving the problem so that the ownership would not be so painful.

The client who displays anger and hostility and who makes unpredictable verbal assaults rarely is the one that staff members flock to visit and care for. Everyone soon agrees that this is a problem to be avoided, or perhaps confronted, but not often accepted as a long-term responsibility. A client who is comatose, requiring thankless time-consuming care, or one whose injury or illness makes the person physically distasteful (burns, overwhelming infections, poor hygiene) evokes pity and concern by care-givers, but again they often are considered part of a day's burden to be cared for as needed and shed as soon as possible. When such a client becomes a long-term responsibility for a primary nurse, however, identifying the cause of the problem and planning the resolution become top priority.

When the heavy part of the case load is physical care, the nurse's aide fits in well for giving the care determined by the primary nurse. However, where the heavy case load is primarily teaching, counseling, and assessing goal achievement or making new goals with the client, the kinds of care-givers needed may be weighted far more heavily toward the professionals. The NCC, obviously, must plan staffing in advance and cannot predict adequately the mix of staff needed on any given unit. Primary nurses and assistants develop a sense of accountability and belonging to "their" group of clients. Disturbing that relationship, even for one day, might be resented and disliked by client and care-giver alike. The NCC, however, has a primary requirement to provide staffing assignments based on the client's nursing needs. That may mandate on a given day a change in assignment of a nurse (not the primary nurse) or an aide to a new and different group of clients than those usually served. When basic physical care needs for one primary nurse's clients are overwhelming, the addition of a nurse's aide can be necessary and welcome; when counseling, instruction, or family intervention are primary requirements for a large group of clients, the addition of a nurse will be appropriate.

The 'Electric Fence Phenomenon'

Our initial experience with permanent care groups tended to promote the "electric fence phenomenon." Because accountability for a given group of clients had been identified, care-givers were reluctant to cross the barrier and respond to other clients' requests or other nurses' needs for assistance. Planning, and communicating the infrequent personnel changes to accommodate client needs, helped cut down on this isolating mechanism and the invisible electric fence disappeared. There are many ways for the NCC to distribute client assignments among the primary nurses, and all have been tried in various settings.

Primary nurses can choose clients according to whatever criteria they wish—medical conditions they feel comfortable working with, age, sex, length of stay, etc. Or a newly admitted client can be assigned to the opening in the primary case load. Or the assignment can be made geographically: each primary nurse has a geographical district consisting of a certain number of beds, and within that area some clients will be their primary clients and some will be primary clients of other primary nurses on other shifts.

Essentially, three nurses share a district for care-giving and divide primary accountability for the clients over the three shifts among themselves. This works well for a number of reasons. Logistically, there is less walking and figuring out where all of one's clients are. There also is less competition among clients if everyone in one area has the same primary nurse. We met clients who compared styles and attention of different primary nurses, particularly if two clients in one room had separate primary nurses. The mix of acute and convalescent care usually was such that a nurse and an aide could provide all the needed service when each district was accepting new clients as others were discharged. The other methods of client assignment do work in many settings, however.

Kinlein, in her book on independent practice, discusses a creative way to provide for autonomous nursing service in a hospital setting.[4] This sounds much like primary nursing, but the way of providing it is different. Kinlein suggests that all clients on entering the hospital be given the opportunity of deciding whether they need and want professional nursing care and, if so, choosing the nurse and agreeing to pay directly for that service.

Kinlein's ideas of isolating the cost of professional nursing care and providing for its autonomy are wonderful innovations; however, there are some problems in this system:

- Since few clients really know what professional nursing can accomplish for them, they would find it difficult to know what to choose, especially at a time when hospital admission occurs. This kind of thoughtful decision is at risk.
- Clients do not know whether they need professional nursing, and the information and assistance needed in this kind of decision would be made better before an acute medical episode intervenes.
- If the client does not opt for professional nursing as a paid service, who will direct the dependent nursing care provided by the institution? And can it be that easily differentiated from autonomous care on a day-to-day basis?

What may happen in such a system is that the best prepared and most competent nurses will not be available to clients. Their service may seem optional, not necessary, and therefore not chosen by clients. It would be better to use Kinlein's idea of a nurse model analogous to the medical one for hospitalized clients, but to acknowledge that both are required and not optional.

Another part of the process that works well is to have the primary nurses choose the assistants or associates who will work with them. This can be done with the available staff on a unit so that everyone is chosen. This serves to commit nurse and assistant mutually to work together.

Uniforms and Caps: Outmoded Symbols?

Primary nursing defines the differences in expectations and practice between professionals and the other nursing care-givers. A common and predictable outcome of this awareness is for nurses then to question the symbols they previously used to define their practice—uniforms and caps. In her initial seminar for our nursing staff, Sylvia Carlson talked about the benefits nurses obtain and the risks they take when they go out of uniform. If nurses really do things differently from nonprofessionals, then that difference should be demonstrable in practice, and uniforms should not be needed to identify a professional to clients. Nurses are nurses because of what they know and what they do, not because of what they wear. This idea can be threatening to nurses who are not at all sure what they do that L.P.N./L.V.N. s do not do, or what it is that clients can identify as professional practice. The benefits are that nurses join the ranks of other professionals, all ununiformed, instead of being seen as another group of task-identified uniformed workers such as police officers, mail deliverers, or the military. Members of the clergy do wear uniforms of a sort, and so do physicians in the clinical setting, but these tend to enhance individuality rather than reduce it. In nursing, the uniform has served to enforce anonymity and sameness, especially when the attire of nursing care workers at all levels of competence looks alike. Other workers also identify with the professional uniform and assume it, and its prestige, for their own. In the hospital where we implemented primary nursing, the dieticians had begun wearing white uniforms and laboratory coats, meaning, as it does in nursing, "I'm part of the administrative clinical staff." Even the admissions office staff and the housekeeping supervisors had gone into white uniforms.

With the advent of primary nursing, members of the professional nursing staff were given the opportunity to go out of uniform and wear a laboratory coat and the name pin for the identification we felt was needed by everyone coming in contact with them. We agreed that clients should be able to differentiate their primary nurse based on the kind of therapy and care they delivered, but others who interacted with nurses might not get to see them in action clinically, so the laboratory coat and name pin were required. Many of the staff immediately took the opportunity; others waited until uniforms wore out and were replaced by civilian clothes. However, nearly all staff members immediately put their caps away permanently. The nuisance, and occasionally the feeling of silliness, that goes with caps made them obsolete overnight. What followed was amusing to watch. The admissions staff began wearing street clothes and laboratory coats. The LPNs lobbied for their own freedom from uniforms, and the desk clerks did the same. The volunteers made known their threefold concerns:

1. They wanted to know how they could assure clients that nurses were in clean clothes if they were not white? They were concerned that nurses now could do their housework and then come in and care for clients in the same clothes. The implied concern was that nurses were persons who needed to be coerced into a uniform, for they lacked the good judgment to come to work in clean clothes.
2. They also were concerned, and rightfully so, that nurses should be identifiable immediately, especially in times of crisis and for families who would want to find them and talk with them. We felt that the identity criteria were appropriate but could be met equally well without the rigid white uniform and cap.
3. They warned that anyone could pose as a nurse and come in and do illegal things to patients. We pointed out that anyone also could easily buy and wear a white uniform and pose as a nurse, too. Our own institution was a good example of the flurry of white uniforms in the many departments, and in the hairdressers and waitresses who visited while still in their white uniforms.

We began to realize that uniforms served as a class barrier in our hospital, and it was a division not complimentary to nurses. This had not been our reason for the change but it became part of the reason for maintaining it.

One of the by then predictable changes in hospitalwide functioning that followed primary nursing implementation was the adoption of the philosophy by others. Housekeeping personnel were directed to their own nursing units, rather than being assigned functionally (waxer, scrubber, etc.) and it was especially rewarding to see how the nursing office quarters took on new polish and organization when we acquired "our" primary cleaning person. The pediatric clients regularly had been a difficult group for the laboratory personnel, but when a special technician was assigned and trained to be effective with children, everyone was much happier. Primary assignments became satisfiers everywhere.

It was not long before the supervisor title began to change in other departments, too. Coordinator became the euphemism for the same old duties in other departments, but comparable changes in function did not occur, as they had in nursing.

SUCCESS GROUP 4: PHYSICIANS AND THEIR NEW POWER BASE

Our work had just begun, because the fourth group involved in the change, the physicians, had many concerns. They demanded much of our energy in proving that what we knew was good for clients and for nurses was good for physicians, too.

The biggest problems for most persons in equating nurses and physicians as coprofessionals are the employee role and lack of primary access from which nurses have suffered. As long as nurses work by the hour for an employer who hires others on an hourly basis, the professional distinction is hard to see. If, added to this, nurses are part of the many services and equipment assigned to rather than chosen by clients, another key part of professional identity is obscured. Physicians on the other hand always have enjoyed those unique identifiers, and corporate medicine still is a dirty word to some. Until recently, corporate nursing was the only kind available, and it was the rare nurse, client, or physician who could see a professional similarity between nurse and doctor.

Physicians have found it convenient and useful to have nurses available in the hospital as part of the services required for providing medical care. In primary nursing, the nurse continues to provide medically directed nursing care, but two other things occur: (1) nurses begin to recognize their responsibility to provide autonomous nursing services as well, and (2) primary nurses are more involved and questioning of the quality of medical care being provided their clients.

Physicians find this bothersome and at the very least are irked and petulant about this added aggravation in their efforts to deliver independent and unquestioned medical care. Many events have brought about the end of the era where physicians were kings and ruled the health care scene unquestioned and alone. Spiralling health care costs and the growing percentage of those costs paid by other than individuals have led to federal government surveillance and direction of medical care. The Medicare and Medicaid legislation in the 1960s made federal and state governments responsible for the medical bills of the aged and the poor. The effective lobbies against high health care costs that these groups never could develop on their own were now, in effect, formed by the government, for they were now the payers of those bills. Government questioned the cost, quality, and quantity of medical care, and began making decisions on what kinds of care were necessary and should be paid. Government also began asking questions about what kind of care was delivered and whether the outcome was effective. No longer were physicians in charge of these activities. The government became the paying client and began setting standards of care for which physicians were accountable.

In these activities, peer review for doctors also was mandated. Companies that insure physicians for malpractice became concerned with their liability as consumer sophistication and demand for quality rose. This concern resulted in skyrocketing malpractice insurance premiums. So, as physicians' care was scrutinized and not paid for blindly, their incomes became threatened; at the same time, they were forced to pay out huge sums to insure themselves for malpractice.

Primary Nursing Becomes a Target

In this state of growing paranoia and anger, nursing, fanned by a growing professional awareness, stepped more forcefully into the health care field and demanded power and decision making for clients. It is far easier for the beleagured physician to blame nurses rather than the government for the state of affairs. Governments are so impersonal, big, and threatening, and they never were friends of medicine anyway. But nurses were a different case, and physicians' anger, resentment, and fear of decreased medical power and money focused easily on them.

Primary nursing is just the framework to invite such an attack. Physicians see nurses as persons to be directed in important medical care activities so that malpractice can be avoided, documentation to assure payment can be made, and the medical status quo maintained as much as possible. Nurses, meanwhile, are questioning the value of the medical status quo. They see physicians as easily the richest paid of the health care workers. They recognize the lack of collaboration with physicians in providing high quality health care, and they are rankled by physicians' lack of understanding of their attempts to deliver autonomous nursing services to clients. The employee status of nurses best assures that their services will continue to be part of the package available to and under the direction of physicians. If clients independently contracted for nursing services, physicians would lose the power or influence over how those services would be provided.

Many of the questioning and demanding activities regarding medical care delivery in which primary nurses become involved are an aid in decreasing malpractice. The medical condition of a client often can change subtly and slowly, and the progression is unnoticed if the nursing caregivers change from day to day. The character of wound drainage, the degree of orientation and alertness, color, and circulation in an affected extremity—all of these conditions can deteriorate and, without recognition and appropriate action by the physician, can result in malpractice liability. Not only does the permanent contact of a primary nurse enhance the possibility of identification of subtle changes, but the ownership that primary nurses feel for their clients also assures that the physician will be questioned and pursued until appropriate care or explanation is given. Obviously, this kind of relationship can benefit physicians in other ways than decreasing malpractice liability. Information from a trusted nurse who knows well the client and the illness conditions will be received and acted on more quickly and thoroughly than when the information flows from an unknown and transient source. Primary nurses can provide both trusted information and subtle but important information, both of which assist the physician in decreasing malpractice liability.

The Swing to Clinical Decision Making

Another strength for physicians in the primary nursing system is that nursing autonomy swings the pendulum toward clinical rather than administrative decision making. The historical triumvirate of hospital administration, medicine, and nursing usually has been weighted toward administration because nursing, in its dependence, reported to that element as employees. With nursing autonomy represented in the triumvirate, the focus of decision making becomes clinical and client centered rather than institution centered. In the pure sense, what is good for clients must be good for the institution that serves them; but sometimes decision making becomes complex and far removed from the clinical scene. Then clients' benefits in any given decision may be subordinated consciously to what is good for institutional growth and profit, or else unconsciously lost in the corporate machinations.

When nursing gains the same autonomy as medicine and administration in decision making in hospitals, the balance will be toward clinical excellence. It is a seeming paradox that as nursing gains autonomy from administration, it gains autonomy from medicine as well, and in so doing strengthens the medical power in that setting. This is accomplished by taking a two-part system—medicine on one side and administration (including nursing as a subordinate adjunct) on the other—and making it a three-part system of medicine/administration/nursing.

In the two-part system, administration supplies nursing service to clients while physicians direct the day-to-day medical activities of nurses. Although there is a split in direction of nursing services in such a system, administration holds the balance of power because it hires, fires, and sets sanctions for nursing care personnel. Administration allows the medical staff to determine the dependent nursing care provided to clients in the institution through doctors' orders and by the setting of standards and policies of nursing care through institutional physician-chaired medical committees, such as medical records, nutrition, patient care quality, discharge planning, pharmacy and therapeutics, and patient education.

The philosophy behind the split nonnursing direction of nursing is that administration knows best how to provide nursing services in a multiservice institution such as a hospital, and physicians are delegated the direction and monitoring of the dependent nursing component. More and more of these nursing elements are being wrested from administrative/medical hands by knowledgeable and political nursing leaders, so that a two-part system becomes three-part and administrative power becomes the minority in the new reallocation. As nursing recognizes and asserts autonomous direction of its unique services to clients, the result is an increase in medical power in an institution.

How the Struggle for Power Evolves

How that happens can be explained in the following way. It must be understood first that both administrators and physicians, when disagreeing on what is needed for care, usually are honestly committed to the client care quality aspect of their alternatives. The differences in approach usually are based on money and on long- and short-term benefits. If there were infinite quantities of money available, there probably would not be any divisions between administration and medical. However, money is finite, and that means available resources can be used only in limited ways. Administrators generally opt for maintaining the fiscal integrity of the hospital and the best possible care, and providing for continuing viability of the institution. Physicians generally opt for the best care now, arguing that only that decision will assure long-term viability of the institution.

For example, physicians will demand that more nurses be hired, preferably those who will follow medical direction, thereby assuring medically directed care will be given promptly, fully, and exactly as ordered. This protects physicians from malpractice and negligence and cuts down on the surveillance visits they must make to clients. Administrators may believe that hiring more nurses is an unnecessary expense and what is needed, instead, is to automate the laundry, or provide for epidemiology service. Both alternatives might cut down on the infection rate and make the hospital a safer place for clients. Physicians argue that they can monitor infections, while in fact more nurses would be the best way to reduce the infection rate.

This power struggle over how to use available funds goes on every day in a hospital. Add to the equation a nursing service dependent on both administration and medicine and those two sides are strengthened a little. Physicians order nurses to provide more frequent care or observation, and administration requires from them more infection detection and better laundry disposal. Clients, however, are the losers since they receive less autonomous nursing care than before because time, like money, is finite and as a result there is less time to identify and treat nursing diagnoses.

If, however, a three-part group were making these decisions, the outcome probably would be different and probably would benefit medicine. Nursing, when freed from medical direction, actually can increase medical power in an institution. To understand this, it is important to see that autonomous nursing service is more complementary and enhancing to medical than to administrative objectives. In the example above, nursing might well opt for hiring more nurses, but not using them for medical surveillance. Instead, it might use its new members to provide more comprehensive identification and treatment of nursing diagnosis. This autonomous service is complementary and helpful to high quality, low liability medical care.

The surveillance physicians might order in a narrow context ("vital signs every two hours," or "change position every two hours") becomes unnecessary in a framework where a comprehensive nursing objective of maintaining optimum circulation is being addressed. Then these medical orders will be included in the nursing plan if appropriate, or the same outcome could be reached in a more comprehensive way. For instance, nursing goals such as the following could be achieved:

Adequate circulation as evidenced by:

1. strong peripheral pulses
2. blood pressure in range 100-120/60-90
3. color pink, including nail beds
4. reddened or broken skin areas absent
5. respirations under 20 per minute and lungs clear by auscultation

Better care of contaminated linen and objective infection control also could be achieved, but not at the expense of numbers of nurses available. In other words, the compromises to obtain better linen and infection control are made somewhere other than in the nursing department. Laboratory functions might be combined to free a person (or hire a person) for infection control, and a more efficient method of providing care for contaminated linen could be achieved with reallocation of personnel in the laundry department.

For too long, new needs have been filled at the expense of nursing. When nursing fills one of the three decision-making chairs in a hospital, direct patient care is less likely to be compromised. This benefits medicine and strengthens its voice in the decision-making process. Medicine may control nursing actions no longer, but it will find that medical care of clients is improved with a complementary professional nursing service than when purely medical direction of an administratively run nursing department was the adjunct for medical care. When nursing assumes the accountability for the health outcome of hospitalized clients, the medical care will be better than when nurses are ordered to carry out tasks within the framework of medical practice. It may be easier now to see how an autonomous nursing service helps improve the power of the medical staff.

Physicians complain that primary nursing is difficult for them because all available nurses no longer know something about all of their patients. Before primary nursing, physicians could be assured of instant response concerning their clients' conditions from any available nurse. With primary nursing, as often as not, the nurse with information about any given client may not be available instantly. The trade-off is that fewer nurses know more about fewer clients. What is lost in breadth is gained in depth. To paraphrase Churchill, "Never have so few (nurses) known so much about so few (clients)." Many physicians must learn the advantages they can gain by working with a nurse who is comprehensively knowledgeable about clients.

Physicians also fight the primary nursing system because they do not understand fully how autonomous nursing service means practicing nursing, not medicine, autonomously. This is especially difficult in the nurse practitioner role. Without a really definite way of stating nursing's uniqueness, there is no realistic expectation that professional nursing will occur. Many important changes in history have been incremental, slow, and steady. In my experience, the change to autonomous nursing, because it is so subtle (and in many ways is similar to medical care) must be a clear, large leap to new practice. Only after the new identity is achieved is true collaboration possible. Without it, working together will mean working for. An analogy might be a child's achieving maturity, making its own way in the world, and then returning to its parents' house to live. This individual has a far better chance of maintaining identity as independent than if the person had remained at home and added on, without bruise or sorrow, the components of independence. Sometimes a rupture is necessary. When we first began our efforts to implement primary nursing, we were assertive, dogmatic, speaking in absolutes, and making many enemies with our physician friends. One asked me five years later, "You're so much softer now and easier to work with. Wouldn't you begin it differently if you had to do it over again?" The answer is no. Without the clear break from dependence, there would have been no autonomy. There are, however, good and bad ways to do it.

Problems of Philosophies and Precedence

There are real problems in primary nursing for physicians, however, and not simply the feared ones just dismissed. The most common ones involve differing philosophies of client awareness and decision making, and who has precedence in determining priority of client problems to be solved by the two autonomous professions.

Nurses are more likely than physicians to give information to clients and share alternatives with them. Part of this is the inherent difference between the two professions, nursing being very much a doing with kind of practice and medicine more of a doing to kind. If nursing is indeed a profession that enhances individual capacity and motivation for health, then the sharing of information and alternatives is vital to legitimate practice. The best possible health status cannot be imposed in the way that a cure can be. For instance, an appendectomy, penicillin therapy for strep throat, or traction for a displaced fracture, all can be relatively successful on a passive, unmotivated client. However, speedy and complete recovery in terms of regaining or improving health requires the client's motivation, concurrence, and assistance. To achieve these ends, nurses share information and choices so that the involvement will indeed be motivating.

Alternatives also are shared because there is no one right way in much of nursing therapy, and goals are individualistic. For example, a client with a heart attack can have bed rest imposed, and, with monitoring, have medications given to prevent lethal arrythmias. When the crisis is over and the client returns home, the exercise, diet, smoking, and general life style changes depend on how much the individual knows about their effects and the motivation for low risk recurrence. Some persons find smoking and a high fat diet offer more quality to their life than the stress and dissatisfaction of limitations for low risk recurrence. Either way, the initial medical treatment and surveillance is the same, but when nursing enters the picture so does the flow of information and choices.

The enhancement of health that nursing offers takes away from its mystique. When a professional service is defined as helping individuals be their best possible selves, this indicates there is nothing particularly unique about it, unlike medicine, which wields fancy instruments in exotic surroundings (operating room) and dispenses magical potions. So the sharing of information and choices, rather than imposing protocols and therapies, makes nursing therapy more open to question as well.

What is helpful, however, is that there is far more compliance with a regimen that has been devised at least in part by a knowledgeable client. Noncompliance with therapy may be far more prevalent in medical treatment just because lack of knowledge and lack of choices breed passivity.

This dichotomy between the ways the two professions work does, however, pose problems for physicians because many decisions for clients are not purely medical or purely nursing, but are a combination. The most common confrontations are in questioning whether to continue or abandon treatment. Particularly when a client is terminally ill, or the outcome of therapy is unsure, nurses and physicians may differ in how much say the client should have in such decisions. Physicians are more likely than nurses to provide therapy in line with the family's wishes, or to avoid the possibility of legal repercussions rather than keep in accord with the clients' wishes. Clients will share with their nurse their wishes for life support and therapy measures, and nurses are more apt to follow those requests. Physicians, following their philosophy of deciding what is best for their clients, may deny them access to information about diagnosis as well as treatment alternatives. These differences in philosophy can cause real problems when nurses clearly become client advocates instead of medically directed personnel.

One example I experienced was a policy decision on expanding visiting time through the supper hour. Nurses (and clients) favored this extension so that visitors who worked until 5 p.m. still could visit before the brief evening visiting hour. Physicians did not favor it. They were very clear about their reason, as voiced by a surgeon: "I make my rounds between 5 and 7 and I can't get my work done if I have to answer questions from the families." It is clear that physicians at times prefer to practice in isolation from the family. Although families most definitely can compromise effective nursing care as well, nurses were proponents of the extension because clients wished it. Nurses are less likely to decide against the clients' wishes that something is in their best interests.

Differences in priority of problem solving for clients also pose problems for physicians (and nurses and clients). The most common controversy is over the client's need for health education and self-care abilities before discharge. Most physicians believe that the costly institutional setting should be used for acute medical crises and that health maintenance should be a Public Health Nursing (PHN) service following discharge. That is true once the client has mastered the skills needed immediately, for PHN service consists primarily of infrequent visits for hands-on care during prescribed workday hours. What also is missing (and rarely reimburseable in PHN service) is the motivational, educational, and counseling support needed to assure long term compliance with new, challenging, and needed health habits. This should be provided with continuity to strengthen the chances of the client's staying out of the acute care setting. Third party payers surely will begin to allow payment for extended hospital stay for health education if it can be documented that such care is indeed associated with fewer acute care readmissions. Again, this is the investment side of health care; it brings a payment in the future.

Physicians also are slow in seeing the immediate benefit of nursing's autonomous role in resolving nursing diagnoses. One physician told me, "all those unhealthful responses will disappear once I cure him and send him home. Anxiety? Of course he's anxious! Pain? It will go. You're wasting your time. Help me with my patient, don't get into all this other stuff. It's simply related to his medical problem." Two things this doctor has not learned: (1) not all unhealthful responses are related to a medical condition; (2) even when they are, the client benefits by having nursing problems resolved concurrently with the medical problem.

Nurses can help best by acting autonomously. One surgeon who was particularly averse to nursing's autonomous role constantly demanded that nursing return to the medical fold. We decided our best strategy was to include him and not fight him. When we gave one of our seminars on primary nursing for another hospital, we asked him to participate and he used his eloquence in our favor. When asked by a visiting surgeon how his clients had fared in the new system, our peer responded: "When I operated on a hernia patient before, I sent him home 100 percent improved; no hernia, no infection, no pain, and with instructions for no heavy lifting. Now, with primary nursing, I send him home 110 percent improved. We accomplish all the above plus the nurse may have identified some other problems, like obesity or excessive smoking, and gotten him on a regime where he's healthier than before the hernia."

Nurses and physicians can work together for a better-than-ever health status for their clients. Primary nursing is a model for accomplishing those goals. To provide for it in hospitals, the nursing staff, physicians, and administrators must:

1. understand that primary nursing is an investment and a marketing device for excellence in nursing care
2. understand that there are clear distinctions between the accountability of nursing and of medicine and provide for their collaboration
3. provide the nursing leadership capable of such development

Provided with this outlook and these strengths, primary nursing can flourish and provide clients with health care that is complementary to the medical care and is an enhancement for optimum health.

Table 4-1 A Comparison of Roles in Primary Nursing

Primary Nurse	Associate Primary Nurse	Assistant Primary Nurse
I. Plans and directs the 24-hour care of clients in unit.	I. Cares for patients over an eight-hour period according to the plan of the primary nurse. In the absence of the primary nurse, takes charge of the assigned unit, directs client care according to the plan of the primary nurse, and directs the work of the assistant(s).	I. Cares for patients over an eight-hour period according to the plan of the primary nurse and under the direction of the primary nurse or associate.
II. Education: R.N.	II. Education: R.N. or L.P.N. II.	II. Education: L.P.N. or N.A. I or N.A. II.
III. Utilizes the complete nursing process in planning and directing patient care.	III. Participates in parts of the nursing process.	III. Participates in parts of the nursing process.
A. Obtains and documents data through observation and interviewing the client and/or family, chart perusal, and health team conferences. Directs data gathering efforts of associates and assistants.	A. Obtains and documents data through observation and interviewing the client and/or family, chart perusal and health team conferences. In absence of primary nurse, may direct the data gathering efforts of assistants.	A. Obtains and documents data under the direction of the primary nurse or associate through observation and interviewing the client and/or family.
B. Diagnoses problematical responses of the client that will hinder a return to or maintenance of health.	B. May make suggestions as to possible problematical responses of client to the primary nurse.	B. Contributes to the primary nurse's formulation of the nursing care plan by providing data obtained while caring for the client.
C. Sets realistic, healthful goals for the client.	C. May make suggestions to the primary nurse for nursing care plan additions or revisions. In the absence of the primary nurse, may add to or revise plan in emergency situations with the	C. Under the direction of the primary nurse or associate, gives general bedside care of assigned clients and carries out selected treatments of clients

approval of the coordinator or nursing supervisor.

D. Plans with the client, family, and other health team members nursing actions to resolve the health problem.

E. Gives or directs general bedside care along with medical and nursing treatments of each client. Assigns elements of care to associates and/or assistants when appropriate. Documents care according to the nursing care plan.

F. Evaluates effectiveness of nursing care in relation to projected client goals.

IV. Recognizes and acts on nursing priorities of care within the unit.

A. Assigns aspects of clinical care according to client condition and competence of associate or assistant.

D. Gives general bedside care of assigned clients and carries out treatments according to medical and/or nursing orders. Documents care according to the nursing care plan. In the absence of the primary nurse, gives or directs care of each client, assigning elements of care to assistants when appropriate.

E. Contributes to the evaluation of the nursing care plan through documentation of client response(s) to nursing therapy.

IV. Recognizes and acts on nursing priorities of care within assigned case load. In absence of primary nurse, establishes priorities of care for entire unit.

A. Assigns aspects of clinical care according to client condition and competence of associate(s).

according to medical and/or nursing orders. L.P.N. documents care according to the nursing care plan.

IV. Carries out nursing care of assigned clients according to priorities established in consultation with the primary nurse or associate.

Table 4-1 continued

Primary Nurse	Associate Primary Nurse	Assistant Primary Nurse
V. Plans and guides teaching of client, family, associate(s) and assistant(s).	V. Follows teaching plan of primary nurse for client and/or family. Teaches assistant when appropriate.	V. Teaches client basic aspects of hospital routine and self care in accordance with the teaching plan and instructions of the primary nurse.
A. Teaches client pertinent aspects of hospital routine, self-care, and health maintenance activities.	A. Teaches client pertinent aspects of hospital routine, self-care, and health maintenance activities under the direction of the primary nurse.	
B. Involves family in the care of the client when appropriate.	B. In the absence of the primary nurse, involves the family in the care of the client as outlined by the primary nurse.	
C. Assists the family in the identification of discharge needs through health care referrals.	C. Teaches assistant aspects of clinical care within job description and competency level.	
D. Plans and guides the teaching efforts of associate.		
E. Teaches associate and assistant aspects of clinical care within their job description, and competency level.		
VI. Maintains effective collaborative relationships with client, family, associate, assistant, coordinator, and other health team members.	VI. Maintains effective collaborative relationships with client, family, primary nurse, assistant, coordinator, and other health team members. In absence of primary nurse, is responsible for positive communication and cooperation between self, assistant, other health team members and the client and family.	VI. Works cooperatively with client, family, and all health team members under the direction of the primary nurse and/or associate.

A. Establishes a one-to-one relationship with the client in which there is open communication and cooperation in identifying and resolving the individual's health needs.

B. Establishes with family a relationship with an active exchange of information pertinent to the nursing needs of the client.

C. Assigns elements of care to associate and/or assistant with fairness, explanation, and supervision.

D. Communicates effectively, both in writing and orally, all pertinent information to coordinator, associate, assistant, or other health team members responsible for client care decisions. Collaborates with other health team members responsible for those decisions.

E. Collaborates with other health team members in client goal setting and problem resolution.

F. Commends effective nursing care of associate or assistant and identifies and corrects nursing care that is below standard.

VII. Supports unit philosophy and maintains standards of client care.

A. Communicates own nursing development needs to coordinator and is

A. Establishes with the client a relationship with an active exchange of information pertinent to the individual's needs.

B. Establishes with family a relationship with an active exchange of information pertinent to the nursing needs of the client.

C. In absence of primary nurse, assigns elements of care to assistant with fairness, explanation, and supervision.

D. Communicates effectively both in writing and orally all pertinent information to coordinator, in absence of primary nurse, primary nurse when present, assistant, or other health team members responsible for client care decisions.

E. Commends effective nursing care of assistants and identifies and corrects nursing care that is below standard.

VII. Supports unit philosophy and maintains standards of care.

A. Communicates own nursing development needs to primary nurse and

A. Establishes with the client an active exchange of information pertinent to the individual's needs.

B. Communicates all pertinent information to primary nurse or associate.

VII. Supports unit philosophy and maintains standards of care.

A. Communicates own nursing development needs to primary

Table 4-1 continued

Primary Nurse	Associate Primary Nurse	Assistant Primary Nurse
receptive to coordinator's assessment of that development.	is receptive to primary nurse's assessment of that development.	nurse and is receptive to primary nurse's assessment of that development.
B. Identifies nursing development needs of associate and assistant.	B. Identifies nursing development needs of assistant.	
C. Promptly identifies areas of inadequate or inappropriate care by any member of the health team and follows appropriate channels to correct the situation.	C. Promptly identifies areas of inadequate or inappropriate care by any member of the health team and follows appropriate channels to correct the situation.	C. Promptly identifies areas of inadequate or inappropriate care by any member of the health team and follows appropriate channels to correct the situation.

NOTES

1. Mary O'Neil Mundinger, "Primary Nurse — Role Evolution," *Nursing Outlook,* October 1973, p. 643.

2. Marie Manthey, et al., "Primary Nursing," *Nursing Forum* IX, No. 1 (1970), pp. 64-83.

3. Dorothy Del Bueno, EdD., Associate Dean of Continuing Education, University of Pennsylvania School of Nursing (1974): personal communication.

4. M. Lucille Kinlein, *Independent Nursing Practice with Clients* (Philadelphia: J. B. Lippincott Co., 1977), pp. 116-119.

RECOMMENDED READING

Carlson, Sylvia, et al., "An Experiment in Self-Determined Patient Care." *Nursing Clinics of North America* V. 4, No. 3, September 1969.

Ciske, Karen L., "Primary Nursing: An Organization that Promotes Professional Practice," *JONA,* January-February 1974.

Marram, G., et al., *Primary Nursing: A Model for Individualized Care.* St. Louis: The C. V. Mosby Co., 1974.

Marram, G., et al., *Cost-Effectiveness of Primary and Team Nursing.* Wakefield, Mass.: Contemporary Publishing Co., 1976.

Fagin, C., "The Public Will Buy What It Wants and Needs." *American Journal of Nursing,* April 1972.

Chapter 5

Nurse Practitioner: More Comprehensive Nursing or Medical Extension?

"By delegating routine medical care to NHPs,* physicians can concentrate their abilities on more serious and complex illnesses, and can extend their services to a much larger group of patients."
Ann Bliss, R.N.[1]

"Just because a nurse carries out an action, that action does not automatically become nursing."
M. Lucille Kinlein, R.N.[2]

The primary nurse and the nurse practitioner both are at risk when developing autonomous nursing practices because of the time and energy needed and the widespread expectation that they will deliver dependent medical care. For the primary nurse, it is the burden of nursing care required as a result of the medical condition and therapy; for the nurse practitioner, it is the extension of medical assessment and care that intervenes as the priority. In each setting, the nurse must have a solid understanding of the professional nursing service that must be added to the medically determined care, and physicians and clients must be shown the complementary value of such service.

THE DIFFICULTY IN MEASURING NURSING ACHIEVEMENTS

Autonomous nursing service is not yet readily identified and valued. Now, in the midst of growing sophistication about medical care, growing concern

---

*NHPs: New Health Professions: nurse practitioners and physician assistants.

107

about mushrooming costs, and growing numbers of health care workers looking for licensure, certification, and autonomy, the nurse practitioner appears on the scene and tries to convince clients (and other purse string holders) that this new service is valuable, cost effective, and necessary to good health.

A new service is more likely to be accepted and valued if it provides a dramatic and immediate change for the good. Mammography, C.A.T. scanners, coronary bypass surgery, and joint replacements all promptly found a place in accepted and valued health care. The dramatic and immediate changes are important in such overnight acceptance; so, too, is the obvious cause and effect relationship between therapy and improved health. All of these ingredients can be missing from an equally valuable therapy—professional nursing. Dramatic, immediate changes occur more often when something is done to a person (medication, surgery), but when the individual treated is an active participant in the therapy, many events occur that prolong and mask the equally valuable achievements. Virginia Henderson's definition of nursing has wide acceptance. A noted nursing educator, author *(Principles and Practices of Nursing)*, and researcher, and one of the most widely recognized nursing theorists, Ms. Henderson believes that nursing's unique function is to assist the individual in the performance of health-achieving activities that the client would perform unaided if the person had the strength, will, and knowledge. In offering this service, nurses provide knowledge, motivational counseling, and the hands-on therapies needed to regain or promote health. In many ways nurses provide the energy or direction for self-help. This probably is the core of nursing at its best.

And yet the paradox: if what nursing has to offer is simply to help me be the healthiest me possible, how can it be that valuable? (I am reminded of a famous quip, "I'd never join a club that would have me for a member.") If nursing could offer something more concrete, it might be valued more highly. Perhaps that is why nurses tend to spend time on techniques and tasks involving machines, instruments, and the mystique of medications. These are visible symbols of a special service.

Nursing also suffers from the fuzzy line between process and outcome. In other words, health achievements are not easily traceable to nursing activity, and therefore the nurse responsible rarely receives credit for change. For example, it is easier to measure and reward a teacher who has taught a child how to read than to recognize and applaud the one who teaches a child to love to read and to learn from the reading. Professional nursing is caught up in the latter example, and suffers for it.

Whenever the client must believe in something enough to carry out the regimen personally, a long time period often is required. Most people today know that cigarette smoking can cause lung cancer. The surgeon who successfully removes a smoker's malignant lung is thanked and rewarded generously for a morning's work. The nurse who, through counseling, sensitivity to special needs, and alternatives, helps a client to forego smoking and thereby reduces the risk of lung cancer's ever occurring, rarely receives the same appreciation, even if the successful campaign took weeks. Preventive services always have the problem of being undervalued because, since nothing bad happened, who knows whether the service was needed? An outcome that is the absence of illness just is not that dramatic. Curing, however, is very dramatic. Health achievements that are incremental and part of a newly internalized life style become what is only natural for a client, who no longer attributes them to superb, motivating nursing care.

The other problem clients have in valuing professional nursing care is that the outcome sometimes is fleeting and nearly always open to interpretation. A nurse practitioner tells of a bedridden client who in one home visit vacillated among three major problems, each camouflaging the other: pain masking anxiety about her dependent state, and anxiety masking deep concerns about problems with her teenage daughter. Although progress was made in addressing these problems, there was no lasting and visible achievement from the nurse practitioner's visit. In medicine, clients are left with talismans to help them believe that therapy has taken place: the incision scar, the bottle of pills. Nursing talismans often are psychological. The nurse practitioner faces these problems:

1. There is frustration involved in trying to measure and demonstrate the outcomes.
2. Competence in professional nursing not only is less visible and measurable but also is harder to achieve than competence in the dependent nursing skills. Since most people tend to do what they are most comfortable doing, autonomous practice is at risk in the inexperienced nurse.
3. The new skills of a nurse practitioner, including history taking and physical assessment, probably were observed most commonly in medical practice, and that is the easiest role to emulate as the nurse practitioner begins practicing.

Clients and collaborating physicians alike expect primary medical care from the nurse practitioner, and it becomes the easiest practice to imitate. Nurses, like other professionals, put on the cloak of appropriate professionalism by watching and working with other practitioners of the same profession. How does one act with clients? How does one approach other professionals? How does one go about the tasks at hand and for what purpose? This assumption of role is an experience that strongly influences the ultimate practice of each individual.

PRIMARY CARE CRITERIA

Nurse practitioners often do not understand autonomous nursing practice before attempting to provide primary care services. When this happens, primary care nursing becomes enhancement of medical care at best, and second class medical care at worst.

This is not an indictment of nurse practitioners. Instead, it is a "cautionary tale" about the pitfalls for clients and nurses if the new role is used to prostitute professional nursing service.[3]

Very simply (perhaps too simply) a nurse practitioner is a registered nurse with special training who can provide primary health care to clients. Primary care is what is requested directly by the client, is comprehensive in nature (diagnosis, treatment, and follow-up from the same primary practitioner), and is directly available, accessible, and accountable to the individual.

In *The New Health Professionals,*[4] Bliss and Cohen describe primary health care as encompassing:

1. promotion and maintenance of health
2. prevention of illness and disability
3. basic care during acute and chronic phases of illness
4. guidance and counseling of individuals and families
5. referral to other health care providers and community resources when appropriate

They add that in providing such services, three elements must be included:

1. all aspects of the individual/family/community such as physical, emotional, social, environmental, cultural, and economic
2. client access to the system
3. a single provider (individual or team) offering continuous coordination and management of basic health care for the individual/family

Bryant, et al., in *Community Hospitals and Primary Care,*[5] define primary care as incorporating one or more of these five concepts:

1. first in time (first contact)
2. usual (repeat contacts)
3. continuing (continuation of care for any given health problem)
4. general (rather than specialized care)
5. health supervision (education and referral)

There seems to be a consensus among professionals and organizational providers concerning primary care components. Primary care has become a fashionable and socially correct goal in health care, partly because of the increase in expensive, fragmented, and episodic medical care. Access and availability to basic primary care have not grown in relationship to the presence of more physicians. The growth of superspecialities, located in preferred urban areas, has been far more apparent.

The federal government is intervening to promote more equitable availability of primary care services. As a result of the Medicare and Medicaid legislation in the mid-60s, the government became the payer of medical care for two large, nonverbal, and powerless groups—the elderly and the poor. These same groups also were in need of medical care more often than the self-insured or those under Blue Cross or Blue Shield. The spotty and often inappropriate care delivered to these minority groups became a primary interest to the government when it began paying the bills. Unnecessary or duplicative medical services were being documented in greater numbers. The idea grew that one responsible (primary) care-giver for each client might cut down on these excesses. The push for national health insurance also had begun again and primary care was seen as the model to assure access to care and proper referral for specialized services.

PRIMARY CARE QUALITY

Both process and outcome of primary care at its best show improved quality as Figure 5-1 illustrates.

When people are treated by an increasing number of specialists, the overall health picture becomes obscured. The one accountable family doctor has gone the way of solo practice into obsolescence. With group practice comes group accountability or, as others have said, "Everybody's business is nobody's business."[6] The return to family practice is a form of primary care. If reports in newspapers and health journals are to be believed, primary care will solve all our ills. It will put caring back into the picture, provide access to and accountability from an identifiable health care provider, be a way of monitoring and evaluating referrals, be a method

Figure 5-1 Primary Care

Process	Outcome
First access	Prevention of illness and disability
Available	Maintenance of health
Accessible	Promotion of health
Comprehensive (diagnostic, treatment, and follow-up with one provider)	Functional assessment (physical, emotional, social, cultural, economic, environment)
Guidance and counseling	Less duplication
Referral	Less unnecessary service
Continuity (health and illness care)	More appropriate use of professionals
	Money saved

---

of providing continuity and comprehensiveness of care, and save money. If more and better service can be provided for less money, it definitely is something to examine closely. The upbeat element is that all the claims probably are true. The greatest likelihood of success in cost-effective high quality primary care may well depend on appropriate use of nurse practitioners. The magic word is appropriate.

Many of the attributes of primary care are available in other high quality models: accessibility, meaning one can reach the source of care directly; availability, meaning that accessibility is available over time; and accountability, meaning the health care provider is answerable to the client for the quality and quantity of care provided. All of these factors also can be present in episodic care, a physician's office, or an outpatient clinic. Continuity, too, may be present, at least for self-identified episodes of illness. In other words, if the client feels ill or notices troublesome or worrisome symptoms, the person can receive care for that complaint (episode).

Episodic care becomes primary care when the person, not just the illness, is treated, and when the detection, treatment, and follow-up come from the same source. A nurse and a physician may offer primary care together to clients; in fact, this is the model that may illustrate primary health care best. The difference between episodic and primary care is a key in determining the outcome. For episodic care, the outcome is resolution of illness; for primary care, it is health maintenance and promotion, a step beyond cure.

Primary means first or most important. Primary care is not referral (surgery, psychiatric, or rehabilitation) but it is a direct access service, such as the family practitioner (nurse or physician) who has direct and regular contact and responsibility for the health status of a group of clients. Primary care implies prevention and maintenance as well as cure. It obviously can take place in a hospital as well as in the ambulatory setting, although it usually begins before hospitalization, when clients choose who will be delivering comprehensive health services, which may or may not include hospital care. Primary care has come to mean ambulatory care to many, probably because it begins and continues most often in the ambulatory, outpatient setting. However, there can be primary care in an institutional setting if the choice of care-giver is the client's and there is continuity, follow-up, and health promotion as part of that care-giver's services.

Primary nursing care differs from primary care nursing. Although the professional nurse in each instance is accountable for diagnosing and treating unhealthful responses and for nursing care planning for an identified group of clients, the similarities end there.

Primary nursing takes place during times of episodic medical care, either during the care or following discharge. Rarely can the client choose a primary nurse and rarely do the acute care responsibilities of the primary nurse allow for follow-up, comprehensive health assessment, and health-promoting intervention. Primary care nursing, on the other hand, demands this initial and complete approach. Primary care nursing is the extended and complete kind of primary nursing. Complete primary health care cannot be provided by either a physician or a nurse alone with the same comprehensive quality that can be assured when the two provide it together. The reason is that both professions offer separate and distinct services, both of which are required for primary health care. There are many skills and services that they share, as well, the most common ones being physical assessment and history taking. Because these two visible activities appear identical, regardless of their purpose or whether they are performed by a nurse or a physician, clients (and nurses and physicians) often are hard put to recognize the difference and the value of joint practice for primary care.

NURSE PRACTITIONER: GENESIS AND IDENTITY

Just what is a nurse practitioner, how does this designation differ from nurse, physician's assistant, or physician, and why did this new category of nurse come about?

It all began at the University of Colorado in the early 1960s under the creative direction of Dr. Loretta Ford, R.N., and Dr. Henry Silver, M.D.

Dr. Ford, with the focus of public health nursing, and Dr. Silver, a pediatrician, worked together on the first pediatric nurse practitioner project. It was a natural outgrowth of Dr. Ford's professional interests at the time, and of national concerns about civil rights, health manpower and widespread access to health care for all. Nursing had gone through a period of specialization where the best practitioners were being rewarded by administrative or teaching positions. The inconvenient hours, poor pay, and dependent status of clinical nursing held little interest for developing professionals. Dr. Ford, among others, was involved actively in looking at what nurses were doing and how better to utilize them clinically. Meanwhile, the civil rights movement and national health insurance proposals were gaining prominence. If all Americans were to receive adequate health care, not only was primary care the best framework, but more comprehensive health care workers would be needed to deliver those services.

The nurse practitioner emerged as an answer to both of these concerns: to provide better clinical utilization of professional nurses and to deliver primary health care to a wider group of persons. This project was meant to use nurses in a wider, more satisfying way, and not necessarily to develop a more autonomous milieu for them. Pediatrics, as the initial area of nurse practitioner development, was particularly productive because so much of child care is within the scope of nursing. It was an appropriate area for this pioneer development. Although children often are ill or injured and in need of medical care, most of their health surveillance and care is centered on normal growth and development. Behavioral, nutritional, social, and physical causes of below-normal growth and development can be diagnosed competently, treated, and managed by a pediatric nurse practitioner. With the advent of that role, more comprehensive health care became available to children, with enhancement of medical care also a part of that service.

Nurse practitioning is the use of better data gathering and the providing of complete nursing care for clients. Many of the differences between nurse and nurse practitioner simply are those in client relationships. With the practitioner, a relationship over time for a variety of conditions and in all settings is possible; in more traditional settings, professional nurse contact is limited to episodes of care, defined more or less by a medical condition. Even in public health nursing, reimbursement stops when a medical condition or at-risk period ends. When reimbursement ends, so does service, so those who decide limits of payment also effectively determine scope of service.

Any nurse can learn the history-taking and physical assessment skills so widely identified with the practitioner role. However, how those skills are used and valued determines whether or not they are part of the usual repertoire of nursing care. If nurses believe that their physical assessment and history duplicate the physician's, then it is easy to see why they do not use these skills. Unfortunately, many practitioners do not understand how those skills differ in outcome reached and therefore tend to use history-taking and physical assessment activities only in lieu of or supplementary to those performed by physicians.

When clients experience nursing without the primary care focus of the nurse practitioner, primary nursing is the most professional model. Primary nurses usually are employees in a given setting, and the client usually is present for medical reasons. Therefore, the professional nursing that is offered is rarely sought by the client, and may be less recognizable and valued because of that. Nurse practitioners are contracted more often by the client for services. Nurse practitioners follow those clients through time, whereas nonpractitioner nurses tend to be part of a package determined by physicians, and the valuable, important nursing care must be fit in around that.

M. Lucille Kinlein, a pioneer in autonomous practice, says of her decision to be called independent generalist nurse:

> The title, "Pediatric Nurse Practitioner" was already in the nursing vocabulary at that time, in 1971. Later, the literature in the nursing field, especially during the years 1973-1975, abounded with articles about the developing movement of the "Nurse Practitioner." In all instances, I found in that movement the same point of departure as in medicine, namely, a frame of reference of pathology; and in most instances there was the need for contact with a physician to varying degrees. I became concerned, therefore, that the title "Nurse Practitioner" would make me appear to be cast in the same mold.[7]

Kinlein is practicing this rather pure form of autonomous nursing. She is using the professional model of access, authority, and accountability to deliver nursing care that is health promoting as well as problem resolving. There is no question that she sees her service as separate and distinct from medicine, both in content and outcome. She has written, "Nursing is assisting the person in his self-care practices in regard to his state of health," which sounds very much like Henderson, and goes on to say, "A nurse can know as much as, and she can know more than, a physician, but she uses the knowledge toward goals of nursing care, which are different from the goals of medical care."[8] At one point in her developing professional awareness she was to exclaim, "I now view medical care as part of nursing care, and isn't that a switch?"[9]

Loretta Ford also recognized early in the practitioner development that the role could be skewed and misdirected toward medicine by physicians, client expectations, and by the nurses themselves:

> Many times Nurse Practitioners act like physician's assistants or like minidoctors or they are caught up in systems that require them to act that way, and have neither the strength nor the understanding of nursing to alter their situation. Nurse Practitioners can not practice in the same way the medical group practices. They have different orientations and goals; they have different expected outcomes. I believe we, as Nurse Practitioners, are engaged in an educative-behavioral model of practice rather than a medical one, if we are practicing nursing.[10]

PHYSICAL ASSESSMENT SKILLS

Primary care nursing most often is visualized as a nurse in an ambulatory setting, taking histories and carrying out physical assessments with all the tools of that trade—stethoscope, penlight, reflex hammer, and a measure of percussion and palpation thrown in as well. Primary care also can be delivered with one's hands in one's pockets.

Primary care is not synonymous with physical assessment. Examples of hands-off primary care are the clients who ask for and require counseling and education to resolve a health problem or lower the risk of one—the new diabetic, the overweight executive, or the stressed and anxious college student. Although physical assessment is not always a requirement of primary care, it greatly enhances the service, especially if the assessment is carried out by the same primary care-giver.

In most nursing care delivery models, the nurse provides service on the basis of the physician's physical findings. Ambulation, prostigmine, and fluid diet all are provided and monitored by a nurse following the physician's physical finding of decreased or inadequate bowel peristalsis. In the outpatient setting, the client with the rales, ronchi, and decreased movement of air in chronic pulmonary disease is provided treatment by the nurse that includes breathing exercises, postural drainage, medication directions and side effects, and counseling on exercise and the danger signs of progressive disease. How much better for the client and that person's relationship with the care-giver if the nurse also were the one identifying and monitoring the physical data pertinent to the health problem.

Most importantly, comprehensive assessment and therapy enriches the client-nurse relationship. Rarely is a client satisfied and motivated by one-way communication, and surely will have questions about the physical findings. In the first instance (decreased or inadequate peristalsis), the client may want to know, "Am I filled with gas?" or "Why am I so short of breath?" or "Am I constipated?" and these can be readily answered by a nurse who can percuss for gas, auscultate for bowel activity, and percuss the level and respiratory movement of the diaphragm. Knowledgeable answers from the nurse practitioner will assure client trust and eliminate some of the hesitancy in following the treatment measures that may be difficult or painful.

If, on the other hand, the nurse would be required to say, "I don't know, I'll ask your doctor," not only is the delay discouraging, time consuming, and demotivating, but it also tends to lower the client's faith in the nurse that knowledgeable care will be provided. In the second instance, the client with respiratory disease may question the effectiveness of postural drainage, and the nurse can percuss and listen to lung sounds before and after the exercise and describe the therapeutic changes to the client. This again is motivating and tends to increase compliance with the prescribed regimen.

Two separate strengths in the nurse's physical assessment skills benefit the client, especially in ways supplementary to the physician's. First it cuts down on the delay of waiting for the physician to be called to provide the needed data. Nurse practitioners are involved legitimately in pathology detection and/or progression, and the magic word is change. Has there been a change in physical findings since the last exam? Nurses are competent in recognizing changing physical signs, especially if they are using physical assessment skills regularly with that client and know the person's normals. In the case of the acutely ill, hospitalized client, changes are assessed and monitored hourly or daily. In the ambulatory case, change may be assessed since the last exam a month or a year ago.

Baselines are the most important data of all in determining the presence of pathology or of its progression. Nurses are not as competent as physicians in diagnosing the specific pathology, but they can be as discriminating in detecting change and can do it sooner than the physician when they are present regularly with a client. When nurses are doing the assessment monitoring, subtle but definitive changes in medical condition can be identified and referred for physician treatment before the client recognizes the need for medical care or medical assessment. The second strength in physical assessment by nurses is that the client benefits by having physical data utilized for health maintenance and promotion as well as for medical care. Physical assessment by the provider of nursing care benefits the client because the findings have different meanings than when used only for pathology detection and resolution. For the nurse practitioner, normal findings signal a whole range of potential health achievements and open the door for nursing therapy to begin. The same normal finding by a physician signals the end of intervention.

USING 'NORMAL' FINDINGS IN PRACTICE

For example, in my practice I saw Sam, a 45-year-old receiving department employee at a local business who had come to our clinic for his first posthospital check-up following his second heart attack. Sam was a robust, talkative, handsome man with a relaxed appearance. His heart rate and rhythm and blood pressure were regular and normal. No other abnormalities were noted and his blood studies all were within normal limits. He reported one incident of tightness in his chest while walking outside in the cold, but otherwise was feeling fine and eating a regular diet, spending most of his time visiting with friends, and was eager to return to work. The physician suggested the use of a 3M mask so he would not breathe cold air, which precipitates angina, told him he could take short walks and return in two weeks. The physician was delighted that the client was experiencing no shortness of breath or pain, that his heart sounded strong and regular, and that his EKG was normal. The medical visit took about 20 minutes and his recovery was pronounced normal.

I spent the next 90 minutes with him, developing his much-needed nursing therapy. Sam related a work situation where his closest coworker "drives me crazy," a home situation where he had postponed his planned marriage "because of this heart thing," and a plaintive comment that "I can't stand to be alone now. I even go visit my sister who I hate just so I can have someone to talk to."

It became apparent that Sam was not handling everything so well after all. He had been told to take his pulse and he had reported a range of 70 to 88 to his physician. He did not know what that meant, or what kind of pulse meant trouble. We talked about when to call the physician for pulse irregularities and about the low and high range of heart rate normal for him. We decided that a warm muffler over his face might be more acceptable than the 3M mask. We talked, too, about what being alone meant for him these days and what he needed to face and think about. He was concerned that he might drop dead as a new husband and therefore had unilaterally called off the wedding plans "until I'm stronger."

I called the physician back in at this point and Sam was assured that his short-term prognosis was good. There were no assurances about reaching 65, but then none of us have those assurances. He said he would try to reschedule the wedding. I asked him if he had resumed sexual activity; first he said no, then immediately said "yes, I have, and you know, my pulse goes up." We talked about the pulse and blood pressure rises and how to go about safe and healthy ways to regain a satisfying and full relationship with his partner. We discussed diet and exercise and developed a routine and progression that was healthy and appealed to him. We also discussed the effect of his coworker on his health, and even the possibility of reassignment. Sam left, seeming relieved by his new knowledge and new decisions. He came back twice, once to tell me smilingly of his reinstated wedding date and once to tell me delightedly that his co-worker had been reassigned. He said he did not "escape" to his sister's any more and that he felt good about the future.

This is an example of normal physical assessment leading to fairly complex nursing intervention. Had there been abnormalities in his exam—rales in his lung fields or an irregular high or low pulse, for instance—Sam would have been the recipient of the highly competent medical care available to him. In that case, the physical assessment findings I elicited would have been used to refer him to that medical care immediately. Both outcomes—medical referral or nursing therapy—are legitimate for nurse practitioner physical assessment.

Although originators of the nurse practitioner role such as Ford and the practitioners themselves such as Kinlein agree on the absolute necessity of keeping the practitioner committed to nursing goals and client achievements, particularly promoting individual health, the current reality is somewhat different. The literature abounds with studies that compare time per visit, use of laboratory tests, and success with compliance between nurse practitioners and physicians. These kinds of studies tend to say that the two do the same thing and therefore are comparable.

Some, perhaps even a majority, would agree with Bliss and Cohen in *The New Health Professionals* that the nurse practitioner arose primarily to meet the need of extended medical care. Bliss and others see nurse practitioners as enhancers and augmenters of medical care extension, and in fact there are strong indicators that practice will continue in this direction. The first and strongest evidence is that although the guidelines of the U.S. Department of Health and Human Services for funding nurse practitioner training programs include the professional nursing activities of identifying and resolving health problems, they also include training for care during acute and chronic illness and management of chronic illness. These last two activities are more easily learned (the medical model is clear and accessible) and easily could take up all of a nurse practitioner's time. Only when health promotion, disease prevention, and health problem resolution are isolated from treatment of illness and disease will both be accomplished. This can happen, and does, when a nurse and physician provide primary health care together, not by interchanging services with each other but by providing the separate and distinct components collaboratively. Detection and management of common diseases and illness are included in nurse practitioner learning programs. This traditionally medical practice always is modified by three guidelines:

1. Initial abnormal (pathologic) findings will be referred to an M.D.
2. Initial treatment for medical care will be offered under direct supervision or through the use of a physician-validated protocol.
3. Management of a stable medical condition will be under the guidance of an M.D., and will be referred back to the physician when any change of condition occurs.

It is this medical aspect that has been most widely identified with the role and makes autonomous nursing care most at risk.

The two questions nurse practitioners must wrestle with in the medical diagnosis and treatment area are:

1. What needed nursing care is being denied my client because my available time with that individual is spent in medical management? In other words, what are the trade-offs?
2. When does medical diagnosis and management really become part of autonomous nursing?

The two always will have gray overlapping areas of practice. For instance, anyone who can read a lab slip can diagnose anemia; measles is measles whether an experienced mother, nurse, or doctor recognizes it; and the same is true of obesity. In uncomplicated cases, the treatment for these conditions can be managed competently by a nurse practitioner. The overlapping areas grow as the knowledge and skill of the nurse practitioner grows. The ability to expand management of common medical problems, however, should not evolve at the expense of nursing care. Instead, the basic and simple medical detection and treatment should be the lesser part of the time and knowledge used by a nurse practitioner. The anemic person may need an iron supplement, but many more elements must be explored and addressed, such as diet counseling, self-assessment steps to be taught (menstrual blood loss, tarry stools), and teaching which symptoms of the cause of anemia must be attended to quickly such as chest pain, fainting, bloody stools, palpitations, or vomiting blood. Unfortunately the notion is widespread that nurse practitioners simply are extenders of medical care and do not have a unique and valuable service to offer.

The New York Times, in an article headlined "Not Nurses, Not Doctors, But a New Breed of Practitioners,"[11] grouped physician assistants and nurse practitioners together as "physician extenders" and said:

> All extenders generally perform similar tasks: screening patients, taking case histories, administering tests. Many diagnose simple illnesses and monitor treatment for chronic conditions, such as hypertension. Serious cases are turned over to a physician, but in practice, the extenders can handle about 75 percent of the patients by themselves.

There is no doubt that nurses can identify and manage common and simple medical conditions. The question, rather, is whether this is appropriate use of nurses considering the range of health services that the public needs. Much of the current research and many of the publications on health status regard medicine as only a partial contributor. In an issue of *Science* devoted to health, two physicians wrote that the most effective means of disease prevention and improved health were other than medical care, and were related more to reducing hazards in the environment, improving nutrition, and adopting healthful personal habits. "The conventional view that physicians must do more or that we must have more physicians certainly misses much of the problem that faces us."[12] And yet of the nation's current health expenditure of nearly $200 billion a year, more than 90 percent is allocated to efforts to control and cure illness, less than 3 percent for prevention, and less than 1 percent for health education.[13] Much of the needed increase in services is in nursing, not medicine.

ILLNESS MANAGEMENT BY THE NURSE PRACTITIONER

Nurse practitioners can learn to diagnose and treat a number of common or predictable illnesses. Other disease states can be managed autonomously or with a protocol and medical validation. A protocol is very much like a botany book used to key plants and essentially is an outline of care to be provided, with choices along the way, depending on findings. Another name is algorithms. Protocols can be developed for symptoms (sore throat) or for diseases (diabetes). Figure 5-2 illustrates a possible protocol for sore throat.

Figure 5-2 Sore Throat Treatment Guidelines

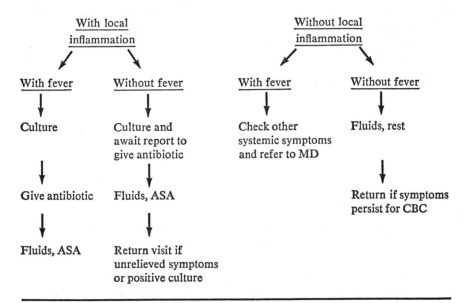

These guidelines, when developed with a physician coworker, can provide excellent assistance in determining therapy and in assuring complete assessment. Nurses can learn to detect and treat diseases autonomously or with the assistance of protocols, and because of nursing's unique competencies, many illnesses are managed more effectively by nurses than by physicians.

The three criteria for illnesses that can be used to invoke nurse management involve situations in which:

1. successful management requires a high degree of client compliance (i.e.: diet, medicines, exercises)
2. teaching, motivation, or counseling are necessary for a cure or for prevention, especially when repeat appointments or learning progressions are needed
3. self-care is the desired outcome

It also is important that diseases meeting these guidelines be fairly stable so that emergency medical intervention is not part of the predictable course of treatment. Myocardial infarction resolution obviously takes a high degree of client cooperation and knowledge, but the acute medical nature of this condition precludes its being managed autonomously by a nurse. However, cardiac rehabilitation, once the risk of recurrence or extension is low, can be a highly effective area of independent activity by a nurse.

Situations that involve the foregoing criteria are such chronic conditions as diabetes, obesity, hypertension, and CVA-deficits, and those slowly deteriorating conditions when they become terminal, such as some cancers, amyolateral sclerosis and concerns of aging such as decreased sight, hearing, and neuromuscular control.

Heretofore, all of these were regarded as medical conditions best managed by physicians. If nurses are to make a formal move in identifying medical conditions they can manage autonomously and competently, and the nurse practitioner movement includes this activity, then they must be responsible and sensible in that choice. To attempt only the diagnosis and treatment of common medical problems is not a legitimate approach. Nurses can learn to identify and treat strep throat (see the previous protocol), but I am not convinced that nurses should be doing this. Every technical hour spent in physical assessment and swabbing sore throats is a professional hour lost in determining health goals or effective compliance with a diabetic or poststroke client. Nurses must move selectively into the medical practice area and take on the management of only those conditions that require nursing therapy as well (including the three criteria already discussed).

Most studies show that clients tend to be more compliant when they see the same professional regularly. In other words, a client being seen alternately by a nurse and a physician will have lower compliance with therapy than when the person sees the same nurse or physician each time. This is another reason for nurses to assume medical management activities in situations where they can provide the full therapy complement. Obviously a physician will be needed often, even with the conditions suggested, for validation of data or therapy (especially when the conditions change), but the actual therapy can continue to be given by the nurse.

Where the needed medical care is received fairly passively without client activity (surgery, casts, radiotherapy), there is little reason to include this kind of management in the nurse's regime. Nothing superior is received by the client in the trade-off; the individual receives the same (or better) treatment if this care remains with physicians. Only when the assumption of medical care by the nurse can show a quality difference for the client should it be done. Too much is being said about giving nurses medical functions if they can do them. There is no question that they can learn many. The issue, rather, is whether the client benefits from that trade-off. It is my belief that the client gets a better deal when nurses manage illnesses that require continuity, teaching, compliance, and self-care.

Advocates of cost effectiveness also must learn that it is not the cost of care (nurses are less expensive than physicians) but the outcome savings that are important. For example, a nurse can indeed detect and treat common infectious diseases such as strep throat, middle ear infections, etc., and will do so for fewer dollars per hour. However, that same nurse could better and more cost effectively be managing a select (chronic stable) group of diabetics, stroke patients, or hypertensives, to keep them well and free of the devastating medical and financial crises that can occur in those diseases with lack of knowledge, skill, or motivation. It is not what nurses can do that should be stressed in this practitioner movement, but what nurses can best do for clients.

Nurses can be selective at this point in determining the kinds of conditions they will manage because there is no void: physicians are managing them. Before taking on the easiest conditions too quickly, nurses must ask some hard questions. The addition of some duties may mean that others will give them up, so that when nurses realize there are other more appropriate areas in which they should be working, there will be no one to whom they can pass the "hot potato." Physicians will have given it to nursing and gone on to perfecting other, probably more complex and interesting areas. The easiest medical activities to assume are the most concrete and most technical, such as throat swabs, pap smears, and infection detection. These probably are not the best areas into which nursing can expand. Rather, nurses should expand into medical areas that they can improve for clients by nursing management.

Other reasons for this thoughtful approach are that the physician assistant is well qualified to take on routine and technological medical activities. Instead of seeing physician's assistants and nurse practitioners as similar extenders of medical care (as Bliss does), nurses must demonstrate their ability to enhance certain areas of illness management, not just to carry out the same existing functions less expensively.

Parkinson's Law tends to occur in health care, also. The amount of work tends to expand to fit the time available. When physicians are relieved of certain duties and nurses take them on, the same work previously done by one physician probably will be done now by one physician and one nurse. Even if there is an increase, it is doubtful that the outcome will double.

THE ENRICHMENT THEORY

Nurses must expand the areas in which they give nursing care, and there are many medical conditions that are better managed by the combined skills of a nurse practitioner than by a physician. If this evolution of a legitimate new practice for nurses is developed using the enrichment theory discussed here, the next step may well be for physicians to expand their practice with some nursing skills to give more comprehensive, health-effective, and cost-effective care. If this were to occur, the difference between nurse and physician in the future might well be defined on the basis of client needs and not simply on their activities. If the client's condition required primarily counseling, teaching, motivation, and self-care, it would be managed by a nurse; if the condition required primarily sophisticated differential diagnosis and complex management and involved mostly doing to (as opposed to doing with) the client, then the physician would be the managing practitioner.

In traditional medicine, therapies are provided more often for and done to the client. Often the condition treated remains a mystery to the client, who simply allows the treatment to be given. Nursing cannot work that way. The client not only must understand the therapies but also must be an active participant and the primary goal setter for personal health. Successful nursing requires the client's assumption of more health promoting and maintaining or curative activities.

This client enrichment theory can be used by nurse practitioners in assuming a wider role in illness management. The practitioner movement is new enough and fluid enough to allow choices of this kind. That luxury will not exist forever. Interim decisions tend to become permanent and many alternatives disappear; expectations become solidified and creative development is stonewalled. Nurses must address this opportunity to expand in nursing expertise for illness management and demonstrate their unique skills. A excellent example of this idea is seen in the hospices. Persons dying of terminal cancer certainly are in the medical illness category, yet because the illness cannot be cured, those so afflicted become very much clients of nurses. Comfort measures, personal care and closeness, nutrition, exercise, and circulation all are in the competent hands of nurses. Narcotic orders and IV fluids can be written as protocols and often are accepted or denied ultimately by the client. The family may become clients of the nurse as well for both physical and emotional care.

Diabetes is another example of appropriate illness management by a nurse practitioner. The kinds of regular assessment needed for a diabetic are blood and urine sugar and ketones, neurologic and circulatory systems, and fundoscopic examination. These assessments can be managed competently by a nurse practitioner. Care should be aimed at an absence of complications and symptoms and toward a satisfied, independent client. Some of the complications and symptoms can be avoided or delayed by proper self-care and compliance with diet and medication. There is no cure for diabetes, and the best outcome is maintaining a high level of health and independence. With the added physical assessment competencies, nurse practitioners also can monitor physiological activity and direct clients showing changes in any of those systems to the appropriate physician.

Physicians have been managing diabetics using the assessment factors listed here and are readily aware of the knowledge, motivation, and self-care competencies such clients require to stay well. However, physicians are not educated in, nor do they have the priority in practice to develop, these client attributes and skills. Nurses do, and nurse practitioner management of diabetics demonstrates well the comprehensiveness of such care.

This idea of nurse management of selected illnesses requires a nurse practitioner. Although that role means a full scope of assessment skills and the ability to function accountably in a primary care practice, the nurse practitioner in practice may not always use both. The nurse practitioner may function in a secondary or tertiary care setting (the hospice is an area of appropriate illness management by nurses) and nurses may not always use the full range of physical assessment skills (psychiatric conditions often do not require extensive physical monitoring). Still, nurses need that range of skills to be legitimately and appropriately ready to manage illness. Instead of the nurse practitioner's being regarded as a new and special breed of health practitioner, skilled in management of common medical problems, that person should be seen as the generic nurse of the future who has extended the scope of client conditions where nursing therapy can be utilized fully. Nurse practitioners must address the components of primary care practice that follow.

AVAILABILITY AND ACCESSIBILITY IN NURSING

Being available means having predictable and identifiable place, time, and equipment to provide services. Accessibility means that the nurse not only is available, but also can be called upon directly by the client to give services and not simply be reachable through organizational screening or physician referral.

Authoritative care means that the nurse has the knowledge and skill to direct comprehensive resolution of health problems and clearly recognizes those for which the therapy is "mine to determine and mine to do."

Accurate care means more than correct or specific—it means also that the data and judgments made are repeatable and predictable by another professional. Whenever service overlaps, there must be concurrence in terms, comprehensiveness, and information between the overlapping professionals. For instance, a grade II/VI heart murmur must mean the same thing to whoever hears it; anxiety must look the same to each professional identifying it (often depression or fear are incorrectly interposed), and negative abdominal examination should mean that each examiner performed the same comprehensive examination and can recognize the limits of normal. Even where therapies differ, as they do between nursing and medicine, the data when duplicated should be identical.

Comprehensive service is a hallmark of primary care. Nurses must have the full range of diagnostic skills to determine the complete nursing therapy needed. Without physical assessment skills and interpretive abilities with selected laboratory studies, nurses would have to rely on others, probably physicians, to give them the necessary data to initiate nursing care. Illness prevention and health maintenance have been included more often in primary care requirements in recent years. Public health practice is grounded in these concepts, and the primary care practitioner is recognizing that they also are requirements in the care of individuals with illness or health problems.

REIMBURSEMENT GUIDELINES

Direct reimbursement for nursing service has been long in coming. The burden for this falls on nurses rather than on organized medicine or on other beneficiaries of the status quo (third party payers, for instance, can deal more easily and economically with just one client—physicians—than with two). There is one acceptable method in which reimbursement now occurs. It combines diagnosis and process: surgery, physiotherapy, hospital stay, sutures, and medication, all have standard reimbursement formulas. Where a physiotherapy payment is the same for each session of therapy, regardless of the diagnosis (muscle spasm from tension or following complex neurosurgery) other reimbursement payments do differ from diagnosis to diagnosis. The most common is the allowed length of stay and reimbursement in hospital.

This diagnosis-process method of defining reimbursement has plagued nursing because, before its unique and autonomous services became articulated, there was no nursing diagnosis, and the process of nursing was seen to be within the direction, liability, and payment of the physician or employing institution. The development of nursing diagnosis will help greatly in obtaining direct reimbursement for nursing services.

Legislation usually follows actual practice; in fact, most of the new nurse practice acts define nursing's autonomy and simply validate and make legitimate the profession's long-standing practices. The same is proving true in nurse practitioner reimbursement, where two colleagues already are receiving direct reimbursement without benefit of specific legislation. M. Lucille Kinlein is being paid on the basis of process. She said, "My clients have supported me in this and said, 'you don't need a doctor's signature for this; this is nursing.' The insurance companies finally came through."[14] The other practitioner, a psychiatric nurse clinician, is receiving insurance reimbursement on the basis of nursing diagnoses developed with the help of the National Task Force on Nursing Diagnoses. She submits her nursing diagnosis, list of therapies performed, and her fee. Just as with Kinlein, the insurance companies paid.

In order to be autonomous, or interdependent, nurses must be able to articulate the problems they solve and the therapies they use. Reimbursement is just another reason to pursue these goals. Without direct reimbursement, there would continue to be the need to ask permission of physicians or employers to perform services or to be paid. It will not work that way.

Direct reimbursement for nursing services will continue to grow if two things occur. First, the articulation of nursing diagnoses and therapy as complementary and necessary to existing documented medical services must be developed. The diagnostic development has a national framework and committed constituency. The related efforts to list, define, and demonstrate nursing therapies are less organized and productive. There are good reasons for this. Most simply, nursing actions seen in isolation from their rationale and outcome usually are difficult to identify as professional. For instance, Blue Cross would be hard put to reimburse for massage, ambulation, or a blood pressure reading as autonomous nursing services. And yet the combination and careful assessment throughout could be done only by a professional if, for example, they were part of initial rehabilitation for a client suffering from a stroke with neurological and circulatory deficits. When, how, for what purpose, and, indeed, whether seemingly simple actions are carried out is the core of professional practice. Therefore, nurses should not denigrate their practice when it apparently is filled with simple and personal care activities for a client. Secondly, outcomes of nursing therapy must be identified and labled. Desirable goals, reached through nursing care, can be acknowledged and paid for.

THE OUTCOME VALIDATES PAY FOR THERAPY

Another colleague, a psychiatric clinician, was deeply interested in the causes of alcoholism. She became interested in the possibility that its root lay in unmet dependency needs. She reasoned that by filling those dependency needs in adult alcoholics, they might be able to regress psychologically and physically to the time in their lives when that deficit occurred. She would give them the nursing care to fill those needs and slowly assist them in growing independently, thereby allowing them to drop the unneeded crutch of alcoholism. Her highly professional practice (knowledge and skill, utilizing nursing diagnosis and planned outcome) consisted for weeks of providing bathing and feeding to hospitalized alcoholic patients. This allowed the dependency needs to be filled in an acceptable way (nurses do bathe and feed sick hospitalized patients) and her hope was that with posthospital counseling and a concurrent decrease in bodily care assistance, they could be cured of alcoholism. She met success in at least one of the five clients she treated. To the uninitiated, the five daily bed baths hardly qualify as autonomous nursing therapy, and to look only at the act was to lose the essence of what really was happening.

This is not an easily solved problem, this identity as a professional based on one's visible therapy. Perhaps the best way to organize the nursing process for recognition as professional is to combine therapy as the sandwich filling between a stated diagnosis and outcome. Therapy then takes its proper place—the core of practice, the very center—and yet validated and recognized as professional when seen in terms of what it resolved (diagnosis) and what it achieved (outcome).

"It ain't what you do, it's how do you do it," and why you do it, that makes the difference. Reimbursement generally is made to the person (or organization) responsible for the care. Obtaining reimbursement really means convincing the payer that nurses are accountable for delivering nursing care. This is the declaration of a profession. Nursing may be the first profession to come to the idea of outcome-based reimbursement criteria. Nurses may do so because the process of their practice cannot be valued correctly in isolation. However, the trend is more and more for outcome-based evaluation of, and payment for, professional practice. PSRO mechanisms and protocols have been developed using discharge criteria (goals) for hospitalized patients. For example, a client should be discharged following appendectomy when the individual meets certain conditions: that the person is afebrile, ambulatory, and has a clean, dry incision. Nursing discharge criteria might be when the same client recognizes signs of fever or inflammation, demonstrates understanding of diet, rest, and activity requirements, and can carry out all ADL independently or has appropriate assistance available.

Obviously, outcome is not enough. Process is important also. If these discharge criteria are not met, then the audit activity goes back to examine the process of care. Perhaps the client was admitted with ambulatory deficits or with an intellectual inability to understand instructions or something in the process of professional care was lacking, such as an unidentified abcess, neglected teaching, etc. When the outcome is not the desired one, as in these examples, the activities require reevaluation. Indeed, even when a desired outcome is achieved, the activities must be monitored. The reason for this is to assess when therapy truly was needed and, when needed, which kind was most effective with the least cost (time, emotion, and resources). For example, when clients do not comply with diabetic self-care, nursing therapy could include any or all of the following:

- physical: assessment on a regular basis
- cognitive: information on the disease, complications, and therapy
- affective: information and counseling on the specific benefits for each individual
- psychomotor: implementation of all the self-care activities needed

The nurse also may go through this teaching repertoire with the family. Some improvement probably will be seen and there will be more compliance than before nursing therapy. However, the same outcome might occur through threat alone ("come back in better shape next month or it's into the hospital with you") or by a better detection of more specific cause of noncompliance (perhaps all that was needed was information on disease process). When nurses become adept at regular goal setting with clients (examples of goals appear in chapter 3, and also form the outcome in the appendectomy case) the nursing treatment modalities that achieve the outcome take on more importance in the eyes of clients and with those paying for that care. Goals or outcomes must continue to be developed. Therapy is goal specific and cannot be seen as a continuing self-important element. For too long, nurses have been satisfied with "support the patient," "let him ventilate," etc., without stating what these activities are to achieve. Nurses must know where they are going in order to know when they have arrived. Goals identify that desired achievement.

CERTIFICATION FOR ADVANCED PRACTICE

Other major issues in nurse practitioner development are certification and deployment. Licensure for nurses continues to follow a minimal compentency test that all R.N.'s take, regardless of the kind of first educational program (diploma, A.D., B.S., or M.S.). Certification has come to mean an advanced competency, or mastery, of certain aspects of practice. Nurse practitioner status can be reached through certificate-granting continuing education programs or through some degree-granting programs. The continuing education programs now are standardized to include four months of classroom instruction and eight months of preceptorship practice. Degree programs that involve practitioner preparation include the same time and content requirements. A certificate for completing either program successfully allows the graduate to practice as a nurse practitioner and to take the American Nurse Association certification examination. The ANA certification no doubt will be the standard procedure for direct reimbursement and in other ways will be similar to passing medical board exams in a specialty. M.D. s and R.N. s take licensure exams, and medical specialists and nurse practitioners take examinations, postlicensure and during their practice, that give them national recognition as specialists in a specific area of practice.

Most of the questions about who should license or certify nurse practitioners have been answered—nurses and nursing organizations will govern the practice of nursing—but how these practitioners are to be evaluated in practice has not been answered.

EVALUATING NURSE PRACTITIONER'S PRACTICE

If practitioners are to be evaluated as medical extenders (decreasing the cost and increasing the access to primary medical care), this will influence the content and success of practice. Because medical extension services are expected from nurse practitioners by most evaluators, and because these are the easiest services for the practitioner to learn and perform, it is probable that that is the practice that will occur. Nurse practitioners with the vision of a more enriching practice with clients—that of professional nursing—may find it more difficult to implement and support. These nurses must demonstrate the complementary and helpful value of their services, rather than their ability to assume basic medical care functions only.

As it stands, nurse practitioner practice is being evaluated in terms of comparing process (how many clients seen a day) and medical outcome (correctness of diagnosis and treatment of common medical conditions) rather than in terms of expanded nursing achievements. This comparison of typical interactions with a juvenile diabetic client illustrates the problems in nurse practitioner evaluation:

A. Juvenile Diabetic: Nurse practitioner medical visit: 30 minutes
   • perform fundoscopic examination
   • perform peripheral vascular and neurological examination

- review blood sugar and triglyceride laboratory report
- take weight

B. Juvenile Diabetic: Nurse practitioner nursing visit: 60 minutes
  - review diet compliance and satisfaction
  - review exercise and social interactions
  - perform fundoscopic examination
  - perform peripheral vascular and neurological examination
  - review blood sugar and triglyceride laboratory report
  - take weight
  - discuss questions and concerns with client and parent

If the nurse practitioner carries out the comprehensive care outlined in example B, only half the number of clients can be seen in one day. If children treated in this manner are more compliant and healthier, and have fewer complications than those treated under the process outlined in example A, is the double time worth it? The answer is obvious, I think, but we do not have such data available, even if this premise is true. Nurse practitioners must begin to develop this kind of proof: that time spent in motivating, counseling, and encouraging people in more healthful self-care is cost effective. Then nurse practitioner evaluation can be on the basis of nursing process and not merely on medical care process. In both of these cases, abnormalities in the physical examination or laboratory findings would be referred to the physician for evaluation.

An actual example of this difference in medical extension and nursing therapy is the case of Van, a seven-year-old Vietnamese girl who appeared in our clinic with what her father described as a "rash" on her arm. Van was .a fragile, beautiful child, quiet, cleanly but carelessly dressed. Her sandal strap was broken and her shoe flopped awkwardly when she walked, and buttons were missing from her dress. On examination, Van was found to have a large, red swollen area on the underside of her left arm near the axilla. It had all the characteristics of a staphylococcus boil. Her axillary lymph nodes were enlarged on that side, her temperature was slightly elevated (100°) and when asked, she acknowledged she did not feel well and that her head hurt. She had no other significant findings except for a large keloidal scar above her left clavicle. The father explained that she had had an infection there following her vaccination in Viet Nam before they came to the United States five years earlier. It occurred to me that she might have had a staph infection then, also, and might indeed be a carrier of that organism. She had no other sores or lesions, no history of recent illness, and her teeth were in fair condition. The physician saw Van, lanced, drained, cultured, and packed the abcess, and gave the father a prescription for penicillin and instructions to return with the child in three days.

Van had been treated compassionately and thoroughly by this very competent physician, and yet her complete health care lasted another hour. I learned from Van's father that he was a student and left her in the care of an elderly neighbor while he attended class in the evening. Van's mother, who spoke no English was, at that very hour, in the opthalmology clinic having minor eye surgery. It is difficult to imagine a more obvious health risk than a fresh eye incision and draining staphylococcus germs in the same small apartment. I called the opthalmologist and he agreed to have Van's mother return to his clinic for dressing changes and care, rather than having her do it herself, at least until the staph infection had been treated adequately. I also spoke with the couple before they took Van home to be sure they understood the need for aggressive cleanliness concerning Van's care and the potential for cross-infection.

I also learned that the father was proud of Van's bravery concerning pain. This encouraged me to stress the extreme discomfort she might be having and I prescribed specific comfort measures as part of the therapy— elevating her arm, fluids, and aspirin. I informed him that although only her arm seemed to be affected, she was indeed sick all over and needed to be cared for as a sick child. For instance, she could not return to school that afternoon so that her mother could rest and her father return to work.

When Van returned for her follow-up visit she was much improved. The culture validated the diagnosis and therapy, and with the packing removed, she was sent home with instructions for her father to soak the wound regularly and redress it. I gave the father a supply of dressings and asked him to bring Van in to see me in three days. When he did so, my original dressing was still in place. I demonstrated how to apply the warm compress, and had him do it for her in the clinic. I called the opthalmologist with Van's progress and successful initial treatment and learned that the mother's incision was healed completely. I arranged for Van to be seen in the dental clinic at a time when her father could take her there and consulted with the physician to follow up on the possibility that she was a staph carrier.

I still was concerned that Van's home environment was not appropriate and asked for a health assessment visit by the public health nurse working in their neighborhood. I asked specifically for her assistance with the compresses, but also included a request for information regarding the family interactions, resources for a healthful environment, and appropriateness of the evening care of Van by a neighbor. I was not sure where the mother went those hours. The report was encouraging: the apartment clean, food and heat adequate, the elderly neighbor a perfect person for Van to be with (the mother worked evenings) and the child was relaxed and smiling.

This kind of extended care took far more time than the medical assessment and care of Van's infection. The best validation for the time spent with this family is that Van's mother's eye stayed uninfected (maintenance), similar future infections for Van may not occur because of dental care and studies to determine and treat her carrier-state (prevention), and the increased comfort and well-being Van experienced as a result of the parental counseling.

Maintenance, prevention, and comfort are difficult to measure as health results, yet this must be an important part of the evaluation criteria for nurse practitioners. The problem inherent in this ambiguous and contradictory evaluation procedure is that it is being done by legislators, financial analysts, HEW personnel, and many other nonnurses who hope to resolve access and cost problems in medical care by transferring simpler medical tasks to nurse practitioners. Evaluation of nurse practitioners' success and productivity should be determined instead by measuring the health status of persons they serve.

PROFESSIONALS DEPLOY THEMSELVES

Medical and federal agency ideas of how to deploy nurse practitioners are paradoxical. The more autonomous one's service is, the less chance that one will be assigned anywhere. True professionals know best what they do, how to do it, and where their services can best be used. Being "assigned" suggests that one is being used for a different purpose; probably to fill the organizational needs of those doing the assigning. This is the biggest reason that nurses are used for nonnursing. Professionals are accountable to clients, not to institutions, or to their organization directors. Once the legal framework for nurse practitioners' practice is well developed, defining activities that they engage in, and reimbursement mechanisms include direct payment to nurses for their services, the likelihood of their being deployed is slim. Bliss describes the unsatisfactory conditions in rural practice that have been responsible for poor access to physicians in those areas and suggests nurse practitioners could practice there: "dispersion of rural patient populations over hundreds of miles of terrain often difficult to travel, the inability of small communities to support a physician, the professional isolation and long hours of rural medical practice, and the sociocultural preference of the M.D.'s spouse and family for urban-suburban living." [15] She adds that if nurse practitioners (and physician assistants) stay tied geographically to M.D. practices (by legislated supervision and reimbursement) the maldistribution of primary medical care will continue.

This may be an excellent theory, but I doubt that the nurse practitioner differs markedly from the M.D. who finds rural practice unsatisfactory because of the long rides over hundreds of miles of terrain, acceptance of low or nonexistent salary, and the isolation, long hours, and lack of social life that physicians' spouses and families have refused to accept. A recent study shows nurse practitioners do, indeed, often choose rural settings,[16] but more because of the autonomy they find there to practice primary health care. If rural populations lack access to medical care, especially emergency technology and assessment and referral of nonemergency medical conditions, then the physician's assistant, not the nurse practitioner, is the traveler-in-the-lonesome-car person needed. Surely the physician's assistant also could refer rural residents to a nurse practitioner if the needs were nursing, such as the noncompliant diabetic, the overweight and tense client who smokes excessively and suffers from chronic indigestion, or the inexperienced, unwed teenage mother. Each of these persons has immediate health needs and preventive care requirements for which the nurse practitioner is the appropriate professional.

Maldistribution and excessive cost of medical care will not be resolved ethically or practically by a transfer of primary medical care to nurses. What can alleviate this national problem is to consider excessive medical fees legitimate only for specialized and required professional medical care. The medical assessment for referral probably can be assumed in rural and underserved urban areas by well-trained physician assistants. Because nurse practitioners learn the same assessment skills does not mean they should use them for the same purposes; because they can identify the need for more extensive medical care does not mean that is how they should be solely utilized.

Those of us who are strong supporters of nurses' practicing nursing know full well the financial and occupational jeopardy we also may be advocating. Physician's assistants with less education and experience already are averaging higher salaries than nurses. Identification with the medical practitioner has let prestige and some of the real gold dust rub off onto the physician's assistant. In the clinic where I work with master's degree nurse practitioner students, the physician's assistant employed there acknowledged that the only difference between him and us was a master's degree— "we do the same thing." At the same time that we learned of his self-declared equality, we found that physicians, when sending clients to the VD clinic run by this physician assistant, address him as "doctor." The first time I heard this, I remarked to the physician that I felt this was unfair and unethical to clients. He said rather shamefacedly, "well, he's more accepted that way."

Coming under the paternal cloak of medicine has important and predictable benefits—support, identification, referrals, and money. Some nurses may opt for those benefits and choose to practice as physician's assistants. If the nurse is identified and functions as a physician assistant, that may be acceptable; however, muddying the waters by having nurse practitioners give dependent medical care in the name of nursing is wasteful and ambiguous, and adds to the maldistribution of health care professionals. This is not a decision of what nurse practitioners can do but what they can do best to serve health needs.

Nurse practitioners should be deployed in the same way that other professionals are—where clients perceive a need for the services and where the practitioners can make a satisfying living attending to those needs. Professionals deploy themselves.

GIVEN OPTIONS, CLIENTS CHOOSE HEALTH CARE THEY WANT

Would-be deployers (notably the federal government) would do well to give clients more say in the health services for which they ultimately pay. Satisfaction so often is a product of choice. People need to know what the full scope of health services includes and what outcome can be expected from each. Professional nursing service must be articulated as a worthwhile investment and not simply an extension of episodic medical cures. The legislation requiring employers with more than 25 employees to offer insurance from Health Maintenance Organizations (HMOs) as well as the traditional Blue Cross-Blue Shield package is a move in the right direction. HMOs survive financially by preventing the need for expensive hospitalization. Professional nursing services are one means to that end.

HMOs MUST BE HEALTH MAINTENANCE, NOT COST CONTROL

Current HMO practices are an attempt to hold down the rising cost of medical care by instituting incentives for providers of care to keep people well. Most HMOs are based on subscriptions by individuals or families for comprehensive care based on a predetermined monthly or yearly fee. All diagnostic and therapeutic care, including hospitalization, is covered by the fee. The HMO survives financially by providing the least expensive care for any given condition. Health maintenance and disease prevention activities should become very important (at least from the provider's point of view) because they keep more of the HMO members out of the risk category of expensive medical care needs. The HMO survives also only by satisfying its members with the care it provides. For example, if hospitalization or access to return visits or tests are denied inappropriately, HMO members will cancel their membership and take their health care dollars elsewhere.

Most people have come to accept, and even expect and prefer, the more expensive forms of medical care. Unnecessary or prolonged hospitalization or surgery, repeat visits for procedures that could be assumed easily by the client (reading tbc skin test results, assessment of minor incision healing, dressing changes, etc.) are costs borne with little objection by many. The passivity in all self-care health practices that this kind of care encourages is destructive. How often we hear the prenatal woman moan, "Oh, my doctor isn't going to like this weight gain," or the diabetic who also places the burden on the physician by saying, "Oh boy, he isn't going to be happy with my blood sugar this month."

In opting for this passive reception of medical (or health) care, the more difficult activities of self-discipline and regular concurrence with healthful behavior can be ignored. And yet, dollars spent on resolution of actual problems incurred from a client's unknowledgeable, careless, or self-indulgent health practices could be used for health maintenance or for achieving an even higher level of health and productivity. People need to be introduced to health care opportunities that provide this kind of educational and motivational activity. Although HMOs certainly are dependent on that outcome (successful self-care activities for health maintenance), the best process for achieving that is not always a part of their service. For instance, nurse practitioners often are employed in HMOs because they can provide, effectively and more inexpensively, basic medical care services such as yearly physical examinations, detection and treatment of minor illnesses, and monitoring of patients returning for follow-up visits.

What is happening in this system is that the same kind of episodic care is being carried on at less cost than before the use of nurse practitioners was instituted. Add to this a more thoughtful and appropriate use of laboratory tests, medications, surgery, and hospitalization, and the HMO practice will provide basic necessary medical care at less cost. However, I believe that client dissatisfaction is built into such a system because there has been little effort to enrich the health care offered while much has been taken away (even if not needed). Rarely is the nurse practitioner functioning appropriately in such a system. We need to expand and raise the quality of health care through use of the HMO concept, but this must include genuine health maintenance activities and not just more episodic medical care.

From an era of passive, dramatic cures at ever-increasing cost, we need now to include the client in the prevention and the therapy and to give more value to maintaining the status quo of good health. This means that effective, client-satisfying HMO practice not only will exclude unnecessary medical care practices but also will have the great plus of individualized health achievements for clients through effective nursing care.

I saw a college student for her yearly physical exam. All the findings were negative. When I asked how she felt about her health, I learned that a few years ago she had given up tennis and skiing because of a knee injury. She felt that her lack of exercise now contributed to her poor diet ("I crave sweets and don't eat much else or I'd really be fat") and increased sense of stress from her studies. She had not had any knee trouble or follow-up care recently. Her range of motion and muscle tone was good and equal in both legs; there was no crepitus or unusual joint rigidity or looseness. She was slightly overweight. I suggested that she begin conditioning exercises and in the absence of any knee pain, weakness, or swelling, she continue the exercises as well as jogging (in proper shoes on a regulation track or campus) for short distances—half a mile to begin with. We revised her diet to include vegetables, fish, and meat as well as sweets. A month later, she was doing well with the exercises, liked her new diet but had not lost weight, and was happy to report that the tension was less. This seems like a simplistic intervention, yet it helped this student carry out some actions she knew she should but for which she had lacked an implementation plan.

These individual interactions are rewarding and valuable, but not enough persons have access to that kind of care to make a lasting impact on group expectations and demands. Unless individualized health services such as these somehow are made available to a wider community, many persons will not know the benefits of choosing professional nursing care as part of their health care.

NEEDED: SHORT-TERM GOALS

Opting for professional nursing means having a stake in the future. So much health-related activity negates the idea that one must pay the piper. Among women, the incidence of smoking is increasing hand in hand with an epidemic of lung cancer. Many Americans are overweight, eat too many fats, and live and work in environments with too much tension and too little exercise. Tomorrow, they say, will never come, the debt will not come due. We are not a nation of self-discipline or deferred pleasures and yet predictable lasting health has a little of each of these components. Sometimes, like children, we respond only to immediate threats, and perhaps professional nursing needs to be defined in terms of immediate benefits and losses, which is difficult to do. Health care strategies must reflect the motivating aspects needed for adoption of healthier behavior.

It is unlikely that future health benefits will motivate people toward different and more healthful life styles if they do not provide immediate payoffs as well. Nurses must help their clients form short-term as well as long-term goals that are motivating and satisfying. Giving up smoking has many benefits, the most dramatic being less likelihood of dying prematurely from lung cancer or heart disease. That may be a sound reason intellectually, but most smokers tend to discount the risk and excuse their habit by saying, "I'll die of something else first" or "smoking is a better vice than the alternatives I have."

The sad story of smoking shows that smokers are not being rational. Another approach is needed. In preventive care, the specter of possible but unexperienced pain, disability, or disease rarely is as effective in motivating healthful behavior as some condition, already present, that the individual would like to be rid of, even if that condition is far less dangerous than the one at risk. In the smoking example, the nurse may find that immediate changes in health will better motivate clients to give up smoking than the long-range absence of catastrophic illness. Such factors include quickly restored respiratory capacity for jogging or tennis; better taste, sweeter breath, and whiter teeth; the probability that they and their children will suffer fewer respiratory illnesses; and more money saved for other healthier pleasures.

Benefits for the Stroke-Disabled

Another group that can benefit enormously from short-term goals are persons recovering from disabling strokes. At one time I worked as a practitioner in a day rehabilitation hospital where most of my clients were elderly and disabled by strokes. My responsibilities included an admission physical examination, referrals to appropriate physicians, social workers, and occupational, speech, and physical therapists; and development of a nursing plan of care. The plan usually included continuing physical assessment to monitor actual and at-risk health problems. The list regularly included these nursing diagnoses:

Ambulation problems related to neuromuscular deficits:
- ataxia
- paralysis
- weakness
- paresthesia
- dizziness

Speech problems related to neuromuscular deficits
- dysarthria
- receptive aphasia
- expressive aphasia

Edema due to decreased ambulation and circulation

Lung congestion related to decreased lung expansion

Decreased ADL related to neuromuscular deficits

Frustration related to dependence, change in self-image, poorly understood prognosis

Depression related to social isolation, dependency, and other changes in self-image

Potential recurrent CVA related to hypertension

Potential hemorrhage related to medication therapy

Our long-term expectations for rehabilitation for many of these people was optimistic and included objectives of independence in ambulation, ADL, and with communication abilities recovered or improved. However, these were considered dreams by many clients because they were so far from those accomplishments. What motivated them best for the exercises and self-care we had prescribed were short-term goals that they usually determined.

We began our initial meeting with each person and the family by asking their expectations of us and what was most important to them. While I most often heard expectations about walking and speaking better, the most important factor to almost everyone was "to be useful again." In many ways they came to us for very specific technical assistance in regaining physical independence, and often that was impossible. If one were to stop here, it would have to be said that we were medical failures with every person unable to progress physically to a more independent state. Yet we were able more often to help them meet that important achievement—to be useful again. Usually we were most successful when we began with a short-term, achievable goal. Sometimes this took the form of "what would you like to be able to do most of all?"

Example No. 1: The Case of Bill

For Bill, who had slept on the couch in the living room since his stroke, that No. 1 goal was to be able to go upstairs and sleep in his bed with his wife. Bill was wheelchair bound because of hemiparesis and his speech was slurred. He was a big man, aggressive and short-tempered, and greatly angered by his physical weaknesses. In the physical therapy department, he was able to learn independent transfers to a straight chair. We had hopes that Medicaid insurance would cover the rental of a stair elevator but the rental company found that the stairway wall in his home would not support the device. We had begun the tortuously slow stair-climbing exercises when Bill surprised us one day with a big smile and the news that he had made it upstairs by lifting himself, in a seated position, one step at a time, with his "good" arm and leg. He was overjoyed and so were we.

Not only was it important that Bill had thought up the successful method, but that he was in charge again, even in such a minor way. For him, the worst parts of his illness were his inability to be master of his own fate and to appear so weak. At one point, when we were being too directive, he railed at us, "I've lost the use of my leg, not my mind." His affected side never did gain strength or use from all our exercises, and his speech remained garbled. He did, however, begin gardening, fixed a broken clock, and, most importantly, went upstairs every night and slept with his wife. He had met his goals if not ours.

Example No. 2: The Case of Anna

Anna provided a different set of circumstances, but again, nursing success was achieved even though her medical condition deteriorated rather than improved. Anna was a beautiful and frail European who suffered a stroke following surgery for an abdominal malignancy. In her sixties, long widowed, and childless, she had supported herself in a rather shabby, genteel way as a secretary. Now she was unable to read ("the words don't make sense") or type, and very aware of her new forgetfulness. She also was weakened from the stroke and the chemotherapy, and was living with a friend nearby so she could visit the rehabilitation center three days a week.

We monitored her physical condition—her blood studies, abdominal examinations, and regular assessment of circulatory, neurological, and mental status. We learned that her friend was being oversolicitous, in Anna's eyes. Most of all Anna wanted a measure of independence and helpfulness in their shared apartment. Making breakfast and lunch was Anna's goal. She was less likely to be forgetful if she felt unpressured in the time she had to do things. Therefore, she planned and prepared breakfast the night before (set the table, filled the coffee pot so that it needed only to be plugged in, sliced and covered the grapefruit) and when her friend left for her job, spent a leisurely time preparing lunch early in the morning.

Anna also wanted to be in charge of her own medication administration, so on the three days she visited us each week she brought her pills and I watched her go about the procedure. Initially she was flustered, forgetful, and completely unreliable. We broke the routine down into steps, with a pill taped to the outside of each bottle and large numbers written beside it so that she knew which pill to take at which hour, and which pill she already had taken. It was a long and frustrating process. She mastered it, but what agony.

Anna was eager to resume typing, hopeful that she could resume a paying job, perhaps at home. The occupational therapist began typing exercises with her. However, we had two major problems: she could not yet recognize written words well and she exacerbated all of her recovery tasks (including typing) by trying to do everything as quickly and perfectly as she had before her illness. So, as she tried to type at a mile-a-minute rate from a manuscript she could hardly comprehend, she dissolved into sobs over the keyboard. We obviously needed a new strategy. Anna had a typewriter in her friend's apartment, and we encouraged her to use it to keep a diary of her self-care and other activities. This way, she was typing from mental not written origin and did not encounter the problems she had in recognizing written words. It also means that her speed necessarily would be slower as she composed the thoughts to be typed. Anna would bring us her diary, and we used it to verify her self-medication regime as well. It was a satisfying activity.

As she made progress in speech therapy (word recognition) her confidence grew and her high anxiety level lessened. Although her stroke symptoms were being managed effectively, her malignancy had spread, and she was readmitted to the hospital for another course of radiation and chemotherapy. In her radiant and selfless way, she expressed thankfulness that her new hospitalization had happened then so that her friend could take a long-planned vacation. Anna never left the hospital.

AUTONOMY AND COPRACTICE

The kinds of short- and long-term health achievements in which nurses are expert in helping clients are indeed an important part of this element called autonomous practice. Because nurses achieve gains autonomously does not mean they achieve them in isolation. Interrelationships with other therapists greatly enrich and enhance the value of nursing care. Nursing care in collaboration with medical care is the most qualitative kind of health care. A term now gaining acceptance in this period of nursing autonomy probably best describes the new maturity of the profession: interdependence. However, that kind of coequality and codependence requires that nursing service be an identifiable component of the comprehensive health care package. Just as adolescence is necessary for maturity, so is nursing's clarion call of autonomy needed in order to move on to the full understanding and provision of health care.

My own understanding of the most comprehensive and legitimate nursing practice is a copractice with a physician, serving a shared group of clients, assessing and treating according to their professionally and self-determined health needs. Clients' needs are not split into medical and nursing areas often enough to validate separate problems. One of the earliest practices of this kind is discussed in a 1967 article by George Reader, M.D., and Doris Schwartz, R.N.[17]

Interrelationships with other than a primary care physician, however, more often are transitory, depending on a specific client's problem. These relationships need updating because of the realization and actualization of autonomous practice in the nurse practitioner role.

PHYSICIAN'S ASSISTANTS AND NURSE PRACTITIONERS

Physician's assistants are the first group of health workers that come to mind because of their newness and apparent similarities to nurse practitioners. The physician's assistant was proposed first in 1961 as "a suggestion to create one or two new groups of assistants to doctors from nonmedical, nonnursing personnel." [18] These groups were but one solution to the problem of shortage of medical-professional personnel in the hospital. Early on, nurses were considered candidates for such service. "By virtue of their educational backgrounds, registered nurses could be trained to engage in specialized programs as physician's assistants." [19] Others suggested "the upgrading of nurses" as physician's assistants.[20] However, both Kadish and Carlson, to their credit, asked whether the ensuing depletion of nurses would be appropriate. The initial paranoic flurry in nursing ("take orders from a physician's assistant? Never.") has mostly subsided. Some "turf" confrontations do occur, and will continue to, because the dependent areas of nursing practice do overlap some of the same activities as those performed by physician's assistants.

Indeed, some nurses are choosing to join the ranks of physician's assistants, for many reasons. The paternal acceptance historically offered by physicians can be very satisfying to some nurses. The borrowed prestige and actual financial gains of close professional association with a physician can be rewarding. Other nurses, mostly nurse practitioners, have taken the physician's assistant examinations in order to meet state certification requirements for prescribing medications, and some nurse practitioner settings require such a service in providing comprehensive health care.

Nurses no longer seem to be responding with wounded egos when they are suggested as appropriate physician's assistant candidates—after all, there is much to learn about the dependent practice of medicine that is not included in the education of a nurse. The continuing and growing issue is the overlap of physician's assistants into nursing practice, particularly in primary health care, and in collaborative practices of nurse practitioners and physicians. Nurses and physicians alike should applaud the idea of a medical assistant who will provide safe, competent, supervised, discrete technological services for clients. This should free the nurse and the physician for their unique professional services.

Unfortunately, physicians who for years delegated nursing care to nurses now are awarding it to physician's assistants. Nurses, having wrested their autonomous functions from the control of medicine, are finding others (physician's assistants) taking directions for similar activities from physicians. Rather than physician's assistants' solving a medical care maldistribution problem (the poor, the rural, the inner city clients), they tend to be distributed along with their supervising physicians both geographically and by population served.

They are taking on the predictable assessment and follow-up activities that nurses use in implementing nursing therapy. For example, a routine physical assessment by a physician's assistant has two likely results—pathology detected and client referred to the physician, or normal assessment with client dismissed. The nurse, in the same situation, would have the same pathology assessment and referral skills plus a far richer alternative for the well client. Nursing enhancement of the well client, already discussed, has little opportunity of happening if physician's assistants (or physicians) are doing routine physical examinations, and there are many good reasons (money, time, duplication, access) why clients will not undergo two physicals—one by the nurse and one by the M.D. (physician's assistant.)

Physician's assistants are being used in primary care settings to manage specific clinics (VD for example) where clients are particularly in need of the counseling and health-promoting services that are uniquely nursing's. They also are being used in institutional settings to monitor medical changes without nurses' understanding or therapy. Pain, fever, electrolyte imbalance, swelling, and dyspnea all have nursing management measures, not just medical therapy, and yet if physician's assistants are doing these interim assessments and monitoring, duplication by a nurse (even though there is a nursing therapy to follow) cannot be legitimized.

At the National Joint Practice Association meeting where nurse practitioners and physicians spoke about their different collaborative practices, one nurse practitioner was asked, "How does your practice differ from the physician's assistant"? The nurse, alas, was at a loss for words. The physician responded helpfully that nurses could do everything that physician's assistants could but physician's assistants could not do all that nurses did. He added that nurses had identifiable autonomous functions whereas physician's assistant functions were entirely within the delegated and dependent realm of medicine. It is obvious that he is one physician who understands nursing.

I think the most legitimate and helpful role for physician's assistants is in dependent medical activities. I do not believe they should be working in primary care or assessment areas, because the nurse with those same assessment skills also has nursing therapy to offer and therefore is the caregiver of choice for those clients.

I think the original idea of a physician's assistant's helping a physician in complex technologies (surgery, casting, dressings) is useful. Physician's assistants can be used in medically underserved areas to offer medical assessment and referral (with well-defined guidelines) and should also be trained to recognize the need for nursing therapy and make referrals to nurses. That probably is asking a lot, since even physicians are not very adept at this.

'ANYTHING YOU CAN DO I CAN DO BETTER...'

However, primary care and management of the chronically ill are far more helped and complemented by nursing intervention than by the physician's assistant. What can nursing do about this risk of maldistribution of physician's assistants? It must demonstrate that it has more to offer. Every time a nurse performs a physical examination (routine or episodic) and dismisses a normal client without assessing and promoting individual health goals, the difference between physician's assistant and nurse practitioner shrinks. Every time a nurse recognizes a health need and calls only for medical assistance without concomitant nursing care, the physician's assistant is an equal alternative. The client in pain, for example, requires more than a narcotic and x-ray; the dyspneic person needs assurance and positioning as well as auscultation and oxygen; the child with strep throat requires more than penicillin.

In the similar gray areas of dependent practice where nurses and physician's assistants both practice legitimately, functions and expectations may be the same but nurses still are accountable (unlike physician's assistants) for identifying and treating unhealthful responses that may or may not be linked to the medical condition. Nurses can do more and they must do those things that show a difference in the quality of the care they provide clients.

The real issue for nurse practitioners in their interactions with physician's assistants is whether they truly can show that difference to clients, because visually, as medical detectives, they look very much alike.

THE WHO AND HOW IN FINDING A NURSE

Interaction with other health care workers changes for the nurse practitioner as well. Many times the identification of the need for nursing will come from another professional. Social workers regularly see individuals and families who present clear indicators of nursing needs. There may be inadequate basic care such as poor nutrition or exercise, or environmental factors such as poor garbage disposal, rats or roaches, overcrowding, or inadequate heat. All of these predispose individuals to health problems and limit severely the maintenance and promotion of optimal health. The social worker also may see unhealthful behavior that nursing care can alleviate or change, such as frustration, anger, depression related to illness or lack of understanding regarding therapy, or unnecessary pain, immobility, or debilitation from similar causes. What happens when these key assessments are made by social workers, or indeed by others, such as physiotherapists, a neighbor, or a physician? Where can they send the client for this nursing care? I do not think there is a good answer today. The only alternatives now are:

1. Public health nursing referral: this is a costly and often ineffective remedy. A public health nurse visit costs about three times as much as a visit to a physician's office. The care often is ineffective because primary care nursing is not the focus of these nurses.
2. Informal contacts with friends or neighbors who are nurses: this kind of intervention usually is delivered free and does not have the same impact or continuity as does an organized, accountable and paid-for service.
3. Referral to a nurse who is in solo practice: these are few and far between everywhere as those available often are in specialty areas (ostomy, psychiatric) because they then are assured more physician referrals because they perform an identifiable function. The generic fee-for-service nurse is not common.
4. Private duty agencies: these generally are nurses hired for a shift of eight or twelve hours in an institutional setting. Some nurses whose services can be contracted through a private duty agency are avail-

able for home visits by the hour, but I know of only one such nurse who is doing this kind of work and who understands autonomous nursing therapy, and her fee is more than double that for a physician's house call. True, the physician could not deliver nursing care at even twice the price, but for clients to choose and accept a new and relatively unknown service (professional nursing) it probably should be available at a fee equal to or below existing health care.

Referrals from other health care providers can be expected only when there is a place to which people can be sent, such as an office or a clinic, or somewhere that a person seeking nursing care can go and find a nurse available to provide care. Referrals, or at least appropriate recognition of who should treat a given problem, will come only when clear and numerous demonstrations by nurses of effective health care are apparent. Until then, most people will see nursing as part of medical care and will seek out doctors to deliver that service, or to delegate it to others.

JOINT PRACTICE: THE INCREMENTAL APPROACH

The best answer to the access problem for nursing therapy probably lies in the development of more joint practices with physicians. Most persons already are in the habit of seeing physicians for nearly all health problems, even the nursing ones. If the physician in such a practice can understand how the division of care would work, and would refer the clients with nursing needs to the nurse, the result would be enormously satisfying to everyone concerned.

When I first broached this idea to an internist, his comment was, "I'm not sure there is enough work for both of us." This was a man who valued the competent physical assessment skills and basic illness management skills of nurse practitioners. What he did not know yet was that they could be used for clients' health benefits in ways other than medical therapy. As I described some common interactions of nurse practitioners that could benefit his clients, he began to see how a nurse practitioner in his practice could mean an expanded health care quality, not a division of existing medical care. He still was not sure that his clients would want to pay for that extra service, and I do not know the answer to that either, but I think some would.

To begin such a service, it almost has to be "free." That is, the person sees the doctor and as an extra, when appropriate, also sees the nurse, who adds to the client's needed knowledge about a disease and/or its treatment. The individual learns alternative and skillful ways to hasten recovery or to keep well, learns what is at risk and how to avoid it, and begins making commitments to future health achievements. On follow-up visits, the client first may see the nurse, who assesses progress on factors they had discussed and who does a preliminary examination that may yield information on those health goals or for the concurrent visit with the physician.

It is up to the nurse to show what can be done for clients that will enrich their health status and to demonstrate to the physician that a nurse collaborator is a marketing plus in the practice. Word of mouth still is the best advertising for professional services. As such a practice develops, the physician understands better what conditions or symptoms are handled best by a nurse, and clients themselves will sort out in their own planning which professional can best attend to a problem.

A Primary Care-Giver in Family Practice

In a family practice, the nurse may be the primary care-giver for concerns such as these:

- child growth and development assessment
- childhood behavior problem treatment
- nutritional and diet assessment and planning
- information necessary for compliance
- skill development needed for compliance
- supportive counseling during accommodation to a chronic illness, acceptance of a permanent diagnosis, changed self-image, transient depression, anxiety, fear, and family and individual bereavement difficulties
- premarital counseling
- family planning assessment and prescriptions
- management of stable chronic illnesses
- routine physical examinations
- complete health histories
- home environment assessments

Physicians will have the potential for expanding the practice by having additional time to focus on areas in which they are most expert—differential diagnosis of pathology and its treatment and evaluation. With a competent nurse and physician engaged in such a joint practice, a qualitatively different service will be offered and in time the word will be out that this is the place for a full range of family health services.

If the client is to receive the professional nursing care as an extra, who pays the nurse during this client orientation and marketing period? The nurse regularly employed by the physician can be a nurse practitioner, who can fulfill the traditional nursing role—assistance with examinations; obtaining information prior to the checkup; assisting clients before, during, and after their visit; even turning on the sterilizer and readying a room if necessary. Obviously, the nurse practitioner is poorly utilized for such services, but the reason is access. In time, the nurse practitioner will be used fully in an appropriate collaborative manner and the unmet technical tasks can be assumed by a medical assistant/technologist of some kind.

I think the nonassertive, working-from-within the traditional role can best assure the effective introduction of this professional nursing service. Many would disagree with me and say that nurses must have faith and pride in their unique service and be willing to take the chance to be sought and paid for their special merit. My innate missionary sense about nursing agrees, but I have been the standard-bearer in enough minor but similar skirmishes to know that solid, incremental, undramatic progress probably is the most lasting. Nurses must believe enough in the ultimate improvement in health care that they can achieve so that they will not worry about the rather colorless method of implementing it. If the function can be introduced as a natural outgrowth of traditional, nonthreatening, and accepted service, it will be more likely to survive.

Identity, the Key to Survival

This seems clearly at odds with the whole premise of this book, which holds that "identity means survival." In primary nursing, the change had to be abrupt and clear. This system involves many nurses, physicians, and significant other persons. Incrementalism can be smothered in the strength of the momentum of the existing system. However, in a one-to-one nurse practitioner-physician team, incrementalism probably is the only change method that will work or be acceptable. The nursing goal, however, remains the same: identity so that necessary and important services do survive. However, identity can develop quietly. The method described here, of enrichment based on existing practice, is far more difficult because the nurse somehow must fit in, add to, or at least minimally change the direction and scope of practice. This kind of incrementalism absolutely demands a clear vision of what the final practice limits should be and what ultimately can be deleted or delegated from the original role in most nursing settings. Usually when one sees the light in terms of what ultimate professional practice should be, one wants to divest the old trappings immediately and embrace the new and better practice. The problem here obviously is that few of us work in isolation, and in every professional practice there is at least one other person (the client) even if there somehow were no coworkers. All nurse professionals, therefore, must go about the work of also changing the vision and expectations of their clients and coworkers in order to assure the survival of their new, improved practice.

Nursing practice, for nurses, can be a major interest. Thought and study lead to the growth of an awareness of the enormous benefits possible for clients through the work of a professional nurse. This promotes a zeal for challenging nursing practice to accomplish these expanded and exacting goals. Obviously, the time-honored nursing rituals begin to look tarnished, overly subservient, and nonthinking. Nurses thirst for the opportunity to really implement these new ideas, new skills, and results, and, in order to do so, are eager to drop those rituals. However, clients are not so quick to make that trade and are suspicious of whether or not they indeed will be the richer for it. My experience has shown that the rituals are very comfortable routines for many persons, who like the idea of having a nurse with whom they feel at ease, who can interpret what the physician is doing, who can be part of the medical routine, and yet who has time for them. For the nurse to play a different, more autonomous, role is unusual, alien, and uncomfortable for many clients. If, however, the nurse is doing recognizable and predictable things, the expanded additional service is accepted easily and happily, and soon is valued and sought. A wise woman once told me, "if you wish to change something, see to it that you continue to conform in the things that are not important so that you will be seen as an acceptable and, therefore, solid, thinking individual." It seems to be good advice, also, for the nurse practitioner who wants to use the new skills and new outcomes. If they can be part of a regularly accepted service, they emanate from a respected and known source and therefore must be good.

Clear Perspective in the Incremental Approach

Another reason for the incremental approach is that it keeps the new skills within the framework of nursing for those who are learning to use them. If nurse practitioners jump into a practice setting where only the new skills are used (e.g., physical assessment), there is less chance that the practice will resemble nursing.

Earlier I noted that the nurse who choses the incremental approach must have a clear vision of where the small steps were leading. If a nurse working in the traditional setting begins to learn the expanded role by acquiring a few of the skills nurse practitioners need, that individual may not understand the grand plan for how the new repertoire of skills fits into a truly nursing role. An example is the nurses in a medical clinic who are taught to take a comprehensive history or who learn chest physical assessment. There is no way they can be expected to use those skills as a basis for nursing care unless their instruction is preceded by a thorough and thoughtful development of the process and outcome of professional nursing. By process I do not mean physical assessment, but rather the nursing process: the methods and rationale of nursing diagnosis, comprehensive and validating data, client-set health goals, a full plan of therapy, and an evaluation of the success in resolving the health problem. Only by pursuing those goals for professional practice will the incremental steps in skill development and implementation make a contribution to improved nursing care.

Too much time is spent talking about the new breed of nurses, their expanded role, new licensure, and certification. What is happening in nursing is happening everywhere. Medical practice is expanding (transplants, new ethical issues requiring new skills and different outcomes), legal practice is expanding (environmental issues, human rights awareness requiring new knowledge and new strategies), the ministry is changing (women as spiritual leaders), and so is teaching (competencies, not just social interaction, are wanted these days). Yet the process of expansion, enrichment, and change is accepted as natural and desirable, and practitioners in those fields are not faced with obsolescence, new titles, or new licensure. One does not hear of the expanded role of the orthopedist or attorney. The reason society has imposed a different, limiting, and nonreciprocal stricture on nursing probably is because that career never has been acknowledged as a free-standing profession that is capable of growth. The struggle over who would certify nurse practitioners is an indication of that point of view.

Perhaps if the nurse practitioner role were acknowledged as simply an expansion of nursing, the incrementalism would evolve quietly and easily. However, too many persons have seen the nurse practitioner developed as an answer to inadequate access and availability of medical care, and that is the seed of the dissension and disorientation among nurses about expanded practice. The most dangerous voices today are those that say "don't spend time and energy deciding what is nursing and what is medicine—just do what is needed for people to make them healthier. We don't need to differentiate medical care and nursing care, we need health care." This is the altruistic sounding hogwash that could be the forerunner of nursing's demise. Not to distinguish nursing's contribution is to lose it. The same is true in the nurse practitioner role. We must keep it bent on achieving nursing results for clients. That, however, is an intermediate goal. Collaborative and combined health care is the ultimate goal. Even so, the nursing components should be as easily recognizable in that service as is the medical component.

AUTONOMY, NOT ISOLATION

Autonomy for nursing means acknowledgment of a unique service. Nurses identify the presence in clients of the need for that service by taking a complete health history, by observing the person, making inferences about responses and behavior, and by using the findings of a physical examination and other data, such as laboratory and x-ray reports. This identification of a need for nursing service is the nursing diagnosis. Nurses also provide the therapy to resolve the health problem identified. Nurses assist the client in developing a health goal, or outcome, that is desirable for that individual, is possible to achieve, and can be aided substantially by nursing care.

Nurses also evaluate the effectiveness of the combined client-nursing activities in reaching the goal. Only when nurses and their clients together can demonstrate and acknowledge these services as uniquely in the realm of nursing can autonomy be claimed. Autonomy means self-directed and accountable directly to clients. Obviously it does not and can not mean working in isolation. Usually autonomy-dependency-isolation concerns arise when comparing or measuring nursing care with medical care. When nursing claims autonomy, this usually means freedom from medical dominance and medical direction. Sometimes, where nurses are employees, autonomy means accountability above and beyond that to the administrator to include primary accountability to their clients.

Autonomy, then, means identity more than isolation. Nursing needs identity and autonomy to survive. However, nursing cannot survive alone in a vacuum. Comprehensive health care requires complementary practice with medicine in service to any client. Interdependence is the end goal for professional development. Nursing is one identifiable slice in the health care pie, it is not the meringue on the medical slice. It stands alone but requires the other services to perfect its contribution. This bakery analogy is a simplistic way of showing the role of nursing in providing health care. It is only too easy, in this period of growing awareness and pride (and resentment) in nurses to overdo their own autonomous identification. To continue this analogy, some want to be a pie all by themselves. This attitude not only will increase the cost of health care, it also will be self-defeating, for nurses need physicians almost as much as physicians need nurses.

The Semantics of Health

It seems to me that health is a subjective assessment. People have their own ideas of when they are healthy. One can, however, feel healthy even if one is diseased (undetected and asymptomatic cancer or arteriosclerosis). But in the absence of disease or pathology, one can be unhealthy. What do all these semantics mean? For nursing they mean that a person can be unhealthy without being in need of medical care. A person who is not able to live a full life (and therefore is unhealthy) may need dietary and exercise prescriptions, identifications of desired healthy behavior that can be achieved through nursing care. Weight loss, muscle-strengthening exercises, stress-reducing regimens, new knowledge for self-care (skin care, constipation resolution through diet), changes for a healthier environment (humidity, noise, privacy), and counseling for more productive familial interactions are examples.

The person who feels healthy (but may have disease) and the one who feels unhealthy (although in the absence of disease) are common and regular occurrences. All need health care. Some primarily need nursing care (the worried well or unhealthy undiseased) and some primarily need medical care (those with disease regardless of their self-assessment of health or unhealth). It seems to me that the assessment of individuals by a professional is required in order to determine the kind of care needed.

This is another reason for suggesting that a nurse and physician work together in a joint practice, as peers, in delivering health care. Nurses who in trying to demonstrate autonomy go into isolated practice (hanging up their own shingle) may. be less effective than the nurse in joint practice. I say this because I do not think clients alone can judge whether they need nursing care, medical care, or a combination. Usually it takes a nurse or physician assessment to determine the nature of the problem and the appropriate therapist to resolve it. To go even further, I think nurse practitioners are competent in assessing both needs—for nursing and for medical care. However, the opposite is not so. Physicians cannot assess the need for nursing care. They generally do not know what it is beyond the dependent nursing activities they direct in the resolution of disease.

The obvious answer, then, is to have nurses make the assessments in a joint practice, referring the medical problems to the physician and keeping the nursing care for themselves. Both the ill and nonill in any such practice eventually will need both nursing and medical services, but at different times.

Does the Rationale Hold Up?

The rationale for a nurse in autonomous solo practice can be questioned for two reasons:

1. The client does not always have the data about presence or absence of disease, and therefore often may self-select the inappropriate health care professional. In other words, the client may present the case to a nurse when it should go to a physician, or vice versa. This tends to prolong the extra visit, extra cost, and fragmentation of care that already is a recognizable problem in today's health care system.
2. Client needs fluctuate between nursing and medical care and often overlap. Having care-givers in different locations presents problems. The client will need to move physically between the two, records will be split, and communication will suffer.

On the other hand, if nurses and physicians offer services separately but together, as is possible, the client receives convenient, comprehensive, collaborative, and complementary care. This can be satisfying, cost effective, and an ideal way of delivering and receiving primary health care. One aspect to be explored in this kind of joint practice framework for delivering autonomous nursing services is how the division of care will be decided— by client or by condition? That is, do certain clients always see the nurse for initial assessments or do certain symptoms of any client determine who sees the individual and provides care on any given visit?

FURTHER ON THE ENRICHMENT THEORY FOR JOINT PRACTICE

In the system I know and like best, the clients belong to both the nurse and the physician, and, depending on their needs, will see either one. Those requiring care for an episode of illness can be assessed (examined) by either professional and appropriate care given. More often than not the physician in a joint practice will continue to diagnose and manage these episodes. Much of nursing therapy takes longer and requires more continuity. Behavioral changes such as compliance, assumption of new health care practices, and obtaining knowledge and skill to maintain or promote health, all take numerous visits and incremental therapies to be productive. Nursing time is better utilized for these kinds of client interactions.

The argument was made earlier that nurse practitioners should be cautious in assuming the technological tasks of medicine—the detection and treatment of simple and limited illnesses such as strep throat, monilial infections, etc. There is a risk that the nurse practitioner could be utilized solely for these duties, leaving true primary care responsibilities (comprehensive health achievements) to others. This is not to say that the new technological skills of the nurse practitioner should not be incorporated into the primary care offered to clients. In other words, in an ideal joint practice where the nurse practitioner has a case load of clients with chronic disease requiring nursing care, those persons may come in at times with a sore throat, a URI, or anemia. It is in the best interests of the client that these limited illness episodes be treated by the nurse practitioner. The argument against the nurse practitioner's assuming the simpler technical tasks of medical practice is meant to assume that they will not do only those things. It is entirely right and appropriate for those services to be part of primary care in a more comprehensive sense.

Although I am suggesting that the best use of nurse and physician, and best service for clients is for joint service by the two professionals, with the care-giver determined on each visit on the basis of the current condition, it also is appropriate for clients to be assigned to one or the other professional for overall primary health care and direction on the basis of long-term health status. For instance, the enrichment theory introduced earlier is based on nurse practitioners as the therapists of choice for illnesses requiring compliance, teaching, and self-care. Therefore, the nurse practitioner in a joint practice may have primary accountability for a diabetic client. When that client develops a limited illness, such as a sore throat, it is preferable for the nurse practitioner to see and treat the individual for that illness, rather than having the person seen by the physician. In another instance, if that diabetic complained of chest pain, the physician would see the client. Not all clients in a joint practice will be assigned deliberately to the nurse or the physician as the primary care-giver. Some will seek care only for illness episodes and not desire or need comprehensive direction and follow-up. Others may be assigned specifically to the physician as primary care-giver, and still others will fit the criteria for illness management by the nurse practitioner.

In a family or a medical practice, the kinds of conditions treated better in a qualitative way by the nurse practitioner also are those that require the most time and continuity. Therefore, clients assigned to the nurse practitioner will be fewer than half of all those in the joint practice. Because of the very nature of nursing and of medicine, time is an unequal need for the two services. Medical conditions more often are physical, more easily recognized, and more definitively resolved. The expertise needed is greater than, or at least equal to, nursing talents but contact time required with the client usually is less. Therefore, an equal division of labor in a joint practice may well look unequal if the number of clients is the factor used to divide workload or to measure effectiveness. Some illnesses or diseases are acquired passively and no amount of education, change in life style, or counseling will affect similar repeat episodes, so extra time beyond providing specific medical therapy is wasted. The physician does the right thing in most instances by seeing many clients in one hour. However, the very nature of nursing is to improve health, which necessarily involves assumption by the client of new information, new attitudes, and new skills. This takes more time than traditional medical therapy, as does valid problem identification. Although there are many baffling medical conditions, and results from tests or assessing change in condition over time do take time, they do not usually require much physician contact time. Nursing care, on the other hand, often requires the presence of the nurse to accomplish problem definition, observation of behavior, and so on.

What this all means is that the client group assigned to the nurse practitioner for primary care may be much smaller than the one assigned to the physician. Whereas effective episodic care by the physician may be provided quickly to a larger group, there may be far more recurrences than when effective nursing care is given over a longer period of time to a smaller group of clients. In other words, the self-care competencies transferred and potentiated in nursing care can have life-long benefits in terms of decreasing medical episodes and expense. Medical care, while often definitively curative, is also given for predictably recurrent episodes of avoidable illness. The economic and life quality benefits in effective nursing therapy more than justify the longer care and fewer clients in a joint practice.

WHO ARE THE OTHER PRIMARY CLIENTS?

As noted, some illness management is qualitatively richer when provided by a nurse practitioner. There are other clients, not ill or diseased, who also should have the nurse practitioner as their primary care-giver. These fall into two categories: (1) the motivated well, and (2) the at-risk well. The motivated well also could be described as the unsatisfied well. These are people who are not ill but are not as healthy as they would like to be. They have low exercise tolerance, poor digestion, tension symptoms, excess weight, etc. The nurse practitioner can do a complete history and physical to assure that there is no disease or dysfunction, then develop, with the client, desired health goals and the therapies to achieve them. Sometimes the motivated well do not start out in that category. They do not identify a need to be healthier. Sometimes it is the nurse practitioner in doing a routine history and physical who elicits or develops client desire for a higher level of health and activity. This is another example of nursing activity that follows the assessment of normal.

The at-risk well are the aged, as well as anyone who has a personal medical history of conditions such as heart trouble or hypertension, or is on medications such as anticoagulants, cortisone, or diuretics that can cause other health problems. The aged are in this category because all disabling health conditions are more at risk with advancing age. Nurse practitioners are particularly suited not only to identify degenerative changes but also to treat clients so that debilitation is halted or slowed. Aging can not be stopped, but many of its sequelae can be lessened through changes in exercise, nutrition, and medication.

Again, some of the same criteria that apply to both the motivated and the at-risk well in determining that the nurse practitioner will be the primary care-giver also determine illness management by the same professional. The requirements are:

1. compliance and recognition of therapy and side effects
2. teaching and the need for more knowledge
3. self-care potential as the goal

Routine histories and physical examinations can be carried out by either the nurse practitioner or the physician in joint practice. My own bias is that the nurse practitioner is the preferred professional for this for two reasons:

1. Nurse practitioners can detect changes from normal and refer only problematical findings to the physician. This saves physician time for the complex differential diagnostic work, referral, or medical therapy initiation. More physician time for the sick is then available.
2. The normal physical examination sets the stage for the nurse practitioner to intervene with the client to manage at-risk situations or to help develop plans for an even higher level of health.

This all sounds fine, but who will pay for this kind of ideal health care? Many of the advocates of nurse practitioners are most desirous of the same care for less money. I doubt that in time nurse practitioners will settle for less money if they are doing "the same thing" as physicians. The better goal is complementary health care whereby the addition of the nurse practitioner provides the client not merely with more of the same medical care but with a different kind of care. Initially, promotive and preventive care is expensive. Those who would not have needed or paid for acute medical care will be paying for preventive care. It will take time to show that payment for professional nursing care is an investment rather than a cost. Perhaps with such care, the incidence of diseases that result from poor or abusive self-care will decrease. With optimal diet, decreased smoking, appropriate exercise, tension-lessening measures, and decreased obesity through nursing assessment and motivation, there can be fewer CVAs or MIs or less cancer. The incidence may stay the same, but the age of occurrence will be older. These are measurable health effects that good self-care probably can accomplish.

The nurse practitioner is the professional best prepared to provide this service. The physical assessment skills to monitor physiological progress toward health goals, as well as history-taking thoroughness to uncover at risk tendencies, are nurse practitioner capabilities that are especially helpful in this kind of health achievement program. If data were available to show how the investment of time and money in buying this kind of health service would pay off in the years to come with less or absent medical disease, the value of the investment would be visible and the public would be more eager to participate and more willing to pay for it.

NURSE VS. NURSE PRACTITIONER

Much has been written here about the special qualitative difference the nurse practitioner can make in clients' health achievements, especially in a joint practice. Nursing still faces a mish-mash of titles and educational preparation, all lumped together under R.N. As clinician, clinical specialist, and now nurse practitioner have arisen within the R.N. ranks, there is more confusion, fragmentation, and concern for the client about what to expect from a nurse. And indeed there is a difference in scope of practice. Nurse practitioner is not a new breed or new health professional as some would have us believe. Nurse practitioner is the generic nurse of tomorrow. The word practitioner was tacked on at a time when the profession and the public needed to identify a big jump forward in the scope of nursing autonomy and accountability. The new skills were a conscious effort to make that giant step, not just incremental progress.

Now that those skills have become incorporated into the practice of many nurses, the differential title is becoming superfluous. As long ago as 1972, almost every baccalaureate nursing program in the country was adding physical assessment skills to its curriculum. Now widespread are master's degree and continuing education programs to teach history taking and physical assessment for baccalaureate degree holders lacking those skills. Management skills based on those data are also being taught.

Eventually every nurse will have the nurse practitioner skills and perspective. Nurse means professional nurse, and regardless of the setting where each practices, the repertoire of skills, the depth and scope of learning, and the accountability to clients for care will be the same.

FOUR CHANGES IN NURSING PRACTICE

Four major changes have occurred in nursing practice to further professional development. All are components of nurse practitioner practice, but have come on the scene over a long period of growth in the profession.

Physical Assessment Skills

First and most visible is the range of physical assessment skills. Nurses always have used physical assessment in their evaluation of patients. The stethoscope has been nursing equipment for decades. However, the full range of physical examination skills, including use of the otoscope, opthalmoscope, and other tools, and percussion, palpation, and systematic observation are new to nursing. The important word here is systematic. The procedure of observation, percussion, palpation, and auscultation, in a predictable replicable fashion, is a hallmark of this expanded nursing practice. Although it is clear that nurse practitioners and physicians may use physical findings in different ways—one to develop nursing therapy to meet health goals, the other to develop medical therapy to resolve illness—the physical findings are identical.

For professionals to be able to use or compare each other's findings, the data should be sought and described in a similar manner. For economy of time and money, either the nurse practitioner or physician can make a physical assessment that then can be used by each profession in its own unique way to establish effective therapy. All professional nurses in the future will undergo nurse practitioner training in this area. Not all nurses will work in primary care, ambulatory settings. Some, if not the majority, will continue to have a regular practice in an acute care hospital or in a tertiary institution such as a hospice, rehabilitation center, or specialty referral hospital. Other nurses will continue practice in schools, public health departments, private duty, or industry.

None of the settings compromises the nursing need for physical assessment skills, either to implement nursing therapy or to alert the client and physician to the need for medical assistance. These skills are time saving, client motivational, and a necessary part of providing and evaluating nursing care. The part these skills play in illness management is well illustrated in medical practice. They are valid also for illness management by nurses, but that is only one of their uses. The emphasis on carrying out the full complement of physical assessment, and in doing it in a predictable routine way, is the new aspect in nursing.

I was asked to demonstrate the physical examination to a group of nurses in a hospital. The education director wanted the staff to learn physical assessment during a six-week course, but my job was to demonstrate the complete examination—the competency for which they all would aim. There is or should be no difference in the manner or content of a physical examination by a nurse or a doctor. Only the aim and content of the therapies will be different. Therefore, the idea that nurses saw something different from what a physician would when they performed an examination was misleading and it seemed inappropriate to give that expectation to these nurses. Nurses have indeed adopted the medical framework in performing physical assessment; after all, the same kind of information is needed, so obtaining it in a predictable way makes sense.

Much has been discussed here about the use of the physical examination for nurses delivering primary care in ambulatory settings. Nurses in other practice areas need the same skills. Those in ICU's and CCUs or in post-surgical or medical units in general hospitals all would benefit from nurses' using these to assess their current or changing condition. I can think of no group that needs this skill more than public health nurses, whose role is discussed more fully later. School and industrial nurses regularly and often are in the position of making initial diagnoses and primary assessments. Injuries as well as insidious health problems may be presented initially to these nurses, who must possess complete assessment abilities, both for referral and immediate or long-term nursing care. The time may come soon when nurses without these skills will be liable for negligent care. Rather than provide a different license for a different scope of practice, it would be safer and less confusing for clients if all nurses had the same competencies.

It has been suggested that nurse practitioners have separate licensure to cover their expanded practice. It appears that clients in any health care setting may require nurse practitioners' skills so how legitimate would it be to staff, say, a school health office with a nurse lacking those skills? Will different licenses really make a difference if clients in both settings have needs for the expanded services? Would it not be negligent, discriminatory, or at the least undesirable, to provide those necessary skills to only one of the client groups?

Probably the most compelling reason for requiring physical assessment skills to be part of the competency of every nurse is because clients may have need for those skills in any setting where a nurse works.

Taking A History: Systematic and Replicable

The second change in nursing introduced through the practitioner movement is history taking. To a lesser extent than the physical assessment
example, history taking for the nurse is similar to the medical process and
content. Whereas physical examination process and findings are the same,
the history taking differs in some important ways. First, the similarities in
a nursing history and a medical history: each is a comprehensive set of
data from the client, family, or records concerning past and present illness,
familial health history, satisfactions, concerns and habits in life style, and
any changes in physical or emotional functioning. As in the physical
examination, it is important to use a systematic and routine method of
obtaining a history so that nothing is omitted and so that findings will be
replicable and may be used by other professionals.

Although nurses have taken histories and physical examination findings
from clients for years, the comprehensiveness and the systematic routine
method are new. The information elicited by the nurse or the physician
can be used by either professional in directing their specific therapy. Therefore, like the physical examination, the findings may be identical but the
aim and content of the therapy different.

More of nursing care will focus on behavioral and educative changes
toward a more healthful life and more of the medical activity will be
directed toward resolution of illness or more specific detection of physiological dysfunction. Because different kinds of information in depth are
needed to determine goals of therapy, history taking by a nurse is somewhat
different. More emphasis is placed on personal interactions, health habits,
and concerns because nursing therapy can make possible more healthful
self-care in clients. Environmental factors, nutrition, and family roles all
impinge on health status, and nurses are uniquely qualified to solve these
problems or to make referrals to alleviate the ones they themselves cannot
solve. For that reason, more information concerning these factors would
be elicited in the history taken by a nurse.

How do clients respond to a nurse's taking their history? Or, for that
matter, how do they respond to the nurse's performing a physical examination? An explanation to the client is in order before either is attempted.
Individuals should know what is going to be done with the information,
and upon learning the purpose, they will be far more cooperative and
certainly less puzzled and hesitant. The way nurses explain their purpose
to clients will influence the kind of information elicited. Clients are told
that information in a history (or from an examination) will be used for
two purposes: (1) to identify any problems requiring medical intervention

by their physician and (2) to identify any areas of at risk medical problems and where health improvements are possible for nursing intervention. The same purposes are true also with the physical examination.

The client might be told: "I am a nurse working with your doctor to provide you with a wider range of health care. I will be taking your history and giving you a physical examination. If I find any changes or problems in your condition, I will have your doctor see you and decide what medical care you might need. I will share with you any problems you might be at risk for, and we can determine a plan to keep you healthy. In addition, we can discuss any areas of your life that you would like to be more healthful such as diet or exercise and develop plans for you to meet some of those goals."

Nursing and clients both have suffered from nurses' traditional incomplete and spotty history and examining skills. It has not been recognized and acknowledged that these functions are necessary for nursing care. Now that the realization is becoming widespread, nurses must incorporate these skills into their practice and implement them in a thorough and methodical way.

At risk situations are the kinds of problems that nurses can prevent but, once they have happened, require medical treatment to resolve. Hemorrhage, stroke, pneumonia, or contractures sometimes are predictable and preventable on the basis of a thorough history and physical, and nursing measures can be instituted to prevent them from occurring. Self-monitoring for early trouble signs is of primary importance. Bleeding gums, easy bruising, and petechiae all signal more dangerous bleeding tendencies. While hypertension is largely asymptomatic, frequent blood pressure readings can be useful. Abdominal pain, nausea, gas, and heartburn all are early indicators of ulcer development.

Nurses can teach their clients the early warning signs and can prescribe preventive activities such as diet, sodium restrictions, medications (e.g., aspirin) to avoid certain potential difficulties. Proper exercise, positioning, support, and nonrestrictive clothing are part of the nursing prescription for someone with leg tiredness and varices. Again, these appear to be simple and perhaps nonprofessional interventions, but their proved effectiveness in preventing drastic medical consequences attests to their worth and necessity.

One approach that often is successful in opening the door at a physical examination is to ask if there is something particular the client wants addressed on that visit. The focus then is on the person's main concern. The client is more likely to give all the information needed if aware from the beginning that the individual's need will be met.

Illness Management as a Part of Nursing

The third factor is illness management. Obviously nurses have been managing illness for as long as they have been taking histories and doing physicals. The newness again is in the autonomy and completeness with which these actions are performed. Illness management requires validation in the detection and concurrence with the treatment by the physician also involved in the case. Given these two elements, the nurse can manage many chronic illnesses by using an agreed-upon medical protocol, providing knowledge, teaching, and motivating new healthful behavior, referring clients to other professionals or services, and working with the family to provide environmental and psychological support.

Nurses' assumption of history and physical examination activities has made chronic illness management possible. These activities had been part of nursing's repertoire long before the practitioner movement arose, but never had there been such a wide range for their use until now. It is to the client's benefit that many more health conditions are available now to nurses for their special services. Previously, clients had nurses available to them only when they were being treated for a medical condition by a doctor. Often the time and opportunity were not available to expand on nursing care needed for those same medical problems. Now clients can seek out a nurse for a health problem and can have nursing interventions provided in conjunction with medical care or alone. The nurse practitioner role has made this possible. For instance, "nursing visits" in out patient departments are becoming routine for teaching, counseling, and assessing chronic illnesses (diabetes, hypertension), and for care of nondisease states (well child care, dietary assistance) as well. Without nurses' primary and initial access, neither they nor clients would be aware of these conditions so no one would know that nursing was needed. It is a lot to ask others to refer clients to nurses' care when many nurses themselves do not recognize the need.

That Primary Care Perspective

The fourth and less measurable change in new nursing practice is the perspective toward clients. Whereas episodic care and technical care were the only frameworks possible to nurses, nurses now can offer services on initial contact for continuing care, encompassing preventive, as well as rehabilitative, services. This complete focus—the primary care perspective —is new for nursing. There now is a sense of accountability for detection and treatment of unhealthful conditions and for follow-up, continuity, referral, and evaluation. There is now a cycle of care rather than an episode. For all the talk in years past about episodic and distributive care, nursing was not in a position to supply anything other than the former. The reasons are many: lack of the full range of skills, lack of primary care settings for nursing practice, reimbursement only for medically directed care, national focus on technological cures and not prevention or health promotion, and recruitment and training for a vocation rather than a profession.

Now that most of these barriers to professional practice are gone, nursing finally can grow by skill development (history and physical examination activities), enlarged scope of knowledge and practice (chronic illness management), and the full cycle of diagnosis, goal setting, treatment, and evaluation. It probably is this last, the nursing process, in the hands of a nurse practitioner that demonstrates the full flowering of professional practice. It also seems to me that every professional nurse should have these skills, this cyclical and complete method of providing and evaluating nursing care, and the primary care perspective: access, comprehensiveness, and accountability. Not every nurse will, or should, practice in a primary care setting. However, each one should have the complete range of competencies for initial, primary, diagnosis, and treatment of a client's health problems, regardless of the setting.

The acceptance of this accountability and expectation is critical for professional nursing to survive. In other words, not only must the unique features of the profession be identified, practitioners also must be eager to demonstrate them and their worth. Nursing only now is ready and finally armed for that kind of endeavor.

Where nursing is now and where it is going in terms of really demonstrating client outcome (and not just nursing content) is similar to where Churchill saw England in 1942:

> Now this is not the end. It is not even the beginning of the end.
> But it is, perhaps, the end of the beginning.[21]

The nurse practitioner may not be the final, best nursing model. It is not yet known whether this is the best framework to enhance and direct therapy for health. But the new skills and new outlook will help further that progress. Strong creative efforts by nurses to build on this beginning are needed now.

NOTES

1. Anne Bliss and Eva Cohen, eds.: *The New Health Professionals* (Germantown, Md.: Aspen Systems Corp., 1977), p. 371.

2. M. Lucille Kinlein, *Independent Nursing Practice with Clients* (Philadelphia: J. B. Lippincott Co., 1977), p. 23.

3. Margaret Olzendski, *Cautionary Tales* (Wakefield, Mass.: Contemporary Publishing Company, 1973).

4. Bliss, op. cit., p. 390.

5. John Bryant, et al., *Community Hospitals and Primary Care* (Cambridge, Mass.: Ballinger Publishing Company, 1976), p. 192.

6. Barbara Stevens, "Why Won't Nurses Write Care Plans?," *JONA*, November-December 1972, p. 6.

7. Kinlein, op. cit., p. 23.

8. Ibid, p. 23.

9. Ibid, p. 24.

10. "An Interview with Dr. Loretta Ford," *The Nurse Practitioner* 1, no. 1 (September-October 1975): 11.

11. Steven Roberts, "Not Nurses, Not Doctors, but a New Breed of Practitioners," *The New York Times*, July 30, 1978, p. E-13.

12. Ernest Saward and Andrew Sorenson, "The Current Emphasis on Preventive Medicine," *Science*, May 26, 1978, p. 893.

13. Jane Brody, "Specialists Look to Preventive Medicine to Improve the Nation's Health," *The New York Times*, May 30, 1978, p. B-5.

14. Katherine Jean Young, "Independent Nurse Practitioner: The Practical Issues of Practice," an interview with Lucille Kinlein, *The Nurse Practitioner*, January-February 1977, pp. 16-17.

15. Bliss, op. cit., p. 373.

16. Judith Sullivan et al., "The Rural Nurse Practitioner: A Challenge and a Response," *AJPH*, October 1978, p. 972.

17. George Reader and Doris Schwartz, "Joint Planning for Patient Care," *JAMA*, Aug. 7, 1967, pp. 364-367.

18. C. L. Hudson, "Physician's Assistant: Expansion of Medical Professional Services with Nonprofessional Personnel," *JAMA*, June 10, 1961, pp. 839-841.

19. Joseph Kadish and James Long, "The Training of Physician's Assistants: Status and Issues," *JAMA*, May 11, 1970, p. 1047.

20. Clifford Carlson and Gary Athelstan, "The Physician's Assistant—Versions and Diversions of a Promising Concept," *JAMA*, December 7, 1970, p. 1856.

21. Winston Churchill, speech at Lord Mayor's Day Luncheon, London, November 10, 1942.

Chapter 6

Community Nursing: Seeing the Forest *and* the Trees

Professional nursing in the community includes assessment and management skills for individual health therapy as well as the far-sighted approach called public health perspective, which measures health status and outcomes in the community, which can be large, such as the inner city elderly, or small, such as a family unit. The nurse works with individuals to resolve health problems, but also maintains a perspective that constantly questions community levels of disease or poor health and the environmental etiologies. A nurse practicing in an ambulatory primary care setting, for example, will see environmentally caused illness (hepatitis, emphysema, fractures) and counsel each individual regarding worsening or recurrence. There also is a primary responsibility to work at the community level for prevention. If hepatitis is traced to local clams, the community nurse plays a responsible role in alerting public health officials, and if more than the predictable number of cases occurred (an epidemic), would provide community education and counseling to large groups of persons about avoiding contaminated seafood, early symptoms, and treatment available.

The community nurse also has a primary responsibility to recognize and identify trends in long-term health problems, such as emphysema, so that appropriate referrals and detection and prevention programs are planned and implemented. Appropriate planning would include requests for data on air quality assessment and industrial compliance as well as implementation of respiratory disease screening and nonsmoking campaigns. Community nurses provide the education, counseling, and screening clinics to detect common health problems in the community and to offer therapy or preventive care.

PUBLIC OR INDIVIDUAL ACCOUNTABILITY?

Another element in community nursing is the overlapping and sometimes conflicting turf for practice. In an institutional setting, a nurse and a physician may have confrontations regarding who prescribes or initiates what treatment, but they agree on the idea of complementary practice and a defined clientele. It generally is agreed also that the institution's employees and attending physician bear the responsibility for providing all of the care for patients while they occupy beds. In ambulatory cases it also is clear that the professional personnel are accountable for medical and health services of individuals who seek care. However, it is not nearly as clear in community health practice who is accountable for what or for whom.

The reason for this in part is that clients generally do not seek out community nurses. In institutional and ambulatory settings, clients come with a specific condition or request for treatment. They have a felt need for nursing care and they have expectations about what they want done and how they expect nurses to fulfill their need. In community nursing, the clients may be identified by the nurse as actually or potentially in need of care. This sometimes is done when nurses providing care in the home to one family member identify health problems in other members who may or may not be receptive to diagnosis or care.

With a student of mine, I visited a young woman with a new baby on a routine home visit offered from the primary care clinic where we work. The clinic cares for people under a certain annual wage on a sliding scale fee, and home visits are made without added charge when appropriate. City taxes fund the clinic deficit. In assessing environmental safety for the baby and socializing opportunities for the young mother, we learned that she worked at home as bookkeeper for her husband, who owned his own tree surgeon business. She is careful to isolate his work clothing, which often is contaminated with insecticides.

When the husband was asked about his own health, he responded that he was "very healthy except for some big lymph nodes." On further examination we learned that for several months he had had several large cervical lymph nodes and that his liver was enlarged moderately. He refused the blood tests and biopsy needed to arrive at a definitive diagnosis, and continued his job without other symptoms. He has returned to the clinic since then for other unrelated episodic visits (back strain) and continues to refuse diagnostic tests. He is an example of the peripheral case finding in which community nurses are engaged regularly, with the common result that many who do not identify health as at risk are not ready to accept care.

The client may be unaware of a need, deny it, not make it a priority, or may fear the consequences. Motivation is much more difficult and complex when clients do not present themselves for care. Just as in psychiatric care, client-felt need is the first and most important factor in effective problem resolving. The combination of a client's perceiving a need for care and therefore seeking help from a nurse (or health care facility with nursing service) makes accountability quite clear: "I have this health problem and I want you to help me. For this service I expect to pay you."

The absence of this situation makes accountability less clear. Is the nurse answerable for nontreatment or referral of real individual health problems? Obviously, when the identified health problem has potential community effects, the nurse is accountable to the community for care and/or referral. If an individual with hepatitis were identified, or if an insecticide factory were spewing unhealthful contaminants into the air, a referral or report would be mandatory. Reporting and enforcement are part of professional accountability to the public. However, an ethical argument rather than a legal issue on accountability arises when an individual's health status is in question but the person poses no threat to others and refuses treatment. Individual freedom to choose and the special knowledge of health professionals meet head-on in terms of "I don't want care" versus "you need care for your own good." Individuals may be only too ready to absolve professionals of responsibility for their health if they choose not to follow those suggestions.

Is there a wider community accountability for nurses so engaged? Many would say even if this were possible it would be undesirable because of human freedom and individual rights. Others would contend that a kind of social contract was involved whereby individuals owed society good self-care since society footed the bill for health problems that were a result of health abuse or neglect.

PUBLIC PAYMENT MEANS PUBLIC ACCOUNTABILITY

More and more health care is financed by public funds for many reasons. Access for all at high quality and at the lowest possible cost means that those who cannot afford or obtain care can be assured of these benefits only by governmental intervention. Self-pay for some (Blue Cross/Blue Shield) and public insurance for others (Medicare/Medicaid) mean inequities, duplication, and a two-class system of care. A national health service plan would try to provide access, excellence, and economy for all, paid for at least in part by public funds. Duplication and inequities will be decreased, as will some of the inappropriate or unnecessary care, as a result of mandated and objective evaluation.

If health care for everyone is paid for increasingly by public money, there becomes a clearer sense of individual accountability to the public for doing everything possible to stay healthy. Take that tree surgeon. Perhaps he has chronic insecticide poisoning, with liver and lymph damage. With prompt diagnosis and treatment, he might not have serious health problems. If allowed to refuse or procrastinate about health care, he eventually might need extensive care totalling thousands of dollars; or he might die, leaving a young widow and child who will need public support to survive.

THE NURSE'S ACCOUNTABILITY TO THE COMMUNITY

In a future health care system that tends toward increased public financing, the community nurse would have an increased community accountability. In addition to the growing conflict between public and individual rights and responsibilities in health care, the community nurse continues to work in the ambiguous accountability structure of current public health nursing practice. As it is now, there is confusion in accountability to the physician for process and to the client for the outcome.

Part of the problem can be traced to the way clients are identified. Those discharged from acute care institutions but still in need of hands-on nursing care and medical surveillance are referred by the attending physician (with nudging from the home care department nurses) to the existing nursing agency in the community that has contracted with the institution to provide these delegated medical duties. Convalescent home care and medical monitoring are carried out by public health nurses and others (nurses and home health aides). Most official agencies are city or county health departments. The nursing services funded are the clinic services for screening and maintenance as well as morbidity or posthospital care. The voluntary agencies usually are religious or are funded through such organizations as the community chest. Fees often are nonexistent or on an ability-to-pay basis for the voluntary agencies. Some fees may be higher because of extensive bureaucratic charges in the public agencies.

The Problem of Reimbursement

Although those agencies are committed to preventive and health maintenance services, there is no per-visit reimbursable charge for a home visit. Home care ordered by physicians for short-term skilled nursing activities is reimbursable on a per-visit basis. For example, a newly diagnosed diabetic will qualify for a few physician-directed visits by nurses who will teach insulin injections, urine testing, and diet. However, if in such a visit the nurse were to identify other health problems in the family (poor nutrition, anemia, depression, inability to cope with child rearing problems, etc.) return calls would not be reimbursable on a per-visit basis unless ordered by a physician and somehow justified as medical care.

Public health departments pay the salaries of public health nursing employees on a contracted basis (i.e., the county and state each may fund 50 percent of the pay of a county nursing agency). All revenues (reimbursed or self-pay visits) are subtracted from the salary amounts due from the state or county. Therefore, public funds pay for nurse-directed visits in a way that does little to increase accountability and that promotes the priority of reimbursable visits. If a county nursing agency, instead, were to give priority status to nursing preventive care visits, the time left for medically directed (reimbursable) visits would be less, and fewer such visits would be made. At the end of the fiscal year, the state and county governments would be asked to pay more dollars in nursing salaries than when reimbursable visit revenues were high.

Governments faced with that kind of increased public funding would hardly rejoice, but would move to eliminate some of the nursing positions in that expensive agency. Even if the autonomous nursing services were more cost effective than the medically directed ones (by keeping at risk people out of hospitals) the measurement and confirming evidence of that cost effectiveness might be years away. Blood pressure monitoring, nutrition counseling, and child guidance all may show up in a population as improved health, but probably not by the end of the year. Again, the problem arises that medical results are more valued because they are quicker, more easily linked to a given therapy, and usually more dramatic. Community nursing, especially its interventions to raise community-wide health status, often is just the opposite of these short-term outcomes.

Bread, Not the Icing on the Cake

A system that subsidizes nursing visits as a lump sum public service maintains the notion that such care somehow is icing on the cake and not reportable in terms of hours spent or goals achieved. In actuality, these nursing visits are bread, not cake, and must be reimbursed and evaluated in the same way. The system covers medically directed home nursing care. Because the official agencies are tax supported, many of the group preventive services such as immunizations, DES screening, lead screening, and family planning are free to the taxed community. Voluntary agencies receive their funds from community contributions and usually are limited to that defined community.

Traditional public health nursing has grown as Medicare has opened the option to paid home nursing care to many home-bound elderly. With hospital costs skyrocketing and evaluation of the appropriateness of hospitalization becoming more stringent, more and more persons are discharged while still in need of regular, hands-on nursing care. In many states, all health insurance policies now must include reimbursed home care services, at least for those discharged from the hospital. Blue Cross, Medicare, and most Medicaid policies also cover needed home care services without preceding hospitalization. This obviously is a cost-effective move if the need is validated because it tends to keep people out of the hospital, and a daily nursing visit may be only one quarter the cost of a daily hospital stay. Therefore, the home care case load no longer includes only posthospital clients but also large numbers of those trying to maintain their health and prevent acute illnesses. This should mean that a greater percentage of nursing visits are nurse directed and consist of highly autonomous nursing services.

Thinking back to the discussion on potential nursing diagnosis, one can see that medical diagnosis at risk is uniquely open to professional nursing therapy, whereas once those diagnoses actually have occurred, the physician becomes the primary therapist. For instance, community nurses can monitor, manage, and treat clients at risk for stroke or myocardial infarction (middle aged or elderly persons with high blood pressure, obesity, or smoking habits, or those with previous episodes of CVA or MI). The nurses can order laboratory reports and interpret them for blood lipids and clotting time. They can perform blood pressure readings, funduscopic examinations, and renal function tests, and obtain and interpret subjective reports from clients. Only when the client has increasing risk, such as new symptoms, decreased functioning, higher blood pressure, or an acute episode of illness, does the physician need to take over as primary therapist.

Even though a greater market for autonomous nursing services can be seen in the community now, the historical and outdated framework requiring medical orders for reimbursed care remains. This changes accountability from the desired health goals as determined by nurse and client to less desirable accountability to the physician for carrying out medically directed activities.

The Role of the Clinics

Another focal point in public health nursing is the clinic, where community health needs are identified and clients present themselves for screening and/or care. These clinics are traditionally tbc, VD, family planning, well child, and immunization. In appropriate geographical areas, lead screening, sickle cell testing, and hypertension screening also are offered. The clinics, when part of an official agency (county or city health department) are funded by the taxes of the inhabitants of that area and their services are free or at a nominal charge to those residents. Other public health nursing clinics are funded by voluntary contributions from a defined geographical or religious community and, again, serve the residents of that area either free or on an ability-to-pay basis. Often these official and voluntary agencies overlap in service area, leaving even more questions as to accountability, duplication, and quality.

Lest any public health nurse read me wrong, let me say that public health nursing services far exceed those listed here, but until expectations and autonomy in all those valuable services are part of the accountability inherent in them, they remain extra and carry little value in describing nursing as it is today.

Payment for public health nursing services is included in most hospitalization insurance. Persons receiving these services often see them as hospital benefits requested by their physician. Payment rarely is directly to the nursing agency. When it is—for those who have no insurance, for example—many persons tend to look only at the tasks of nursing and are aghast at the cost. The assessment that goes unseen with the busy hands of a professional nurse is difficult indeed for the client to recognize, for even with identification of progress or new problems, it ultimately is the physician who will direct major changes in care.

PUBLIC HEALTH NURSING: THE HIDDEN RICHNESS

Many nurses choose the community as one of the few settings in which to practice autonomously and to incorporate teaching and counseling into their client therapy. Those who find satisfaction in these areas have learned they must be creative and clever in order to use their professional skills. Everyone involved in a professional milieu of any kind knows the political behavior that enhances success. Nurses are no different from other professionals in this. The wiles and strategies required for successful nursing access and therapy probably are the same as for any professional working on overlapping turf—social workers and psychologists or social biologists and anthropologists. The difference with this new argument on nursing vs. medical turf is that it represents an enormous change in attitude about nursing. The historical perspective on nursing assertiveness (or lack of it!) makes this new political endeavor more difficult.

Although public health nursing has needed creative practitioners to pioneer in providing independent nursing assessment, diagnosis, and therapies for clients who were supposed to be receiving only medically directed treatment, the time is past when that alone is sufficient. Being able to perform the tasks and fit them into one's schedule is not enough. There must be clear expectation from and accountability to clients for these nursing activities.

A national plan for health care is coming. With it surely will come definitive guidelines for who does what, which means who gets paid for what. If physician's assistants now are licensed for routine history and physical examination activities, common disease management, and prescribing of medications, and if college trained health educators market themselves as the ones to identify and give health education to clients, where will nurses be if their activities in both of these areas have been sub rosa, uncontracted for, unpaid, unevaluated, and probably even unidentified? If nurses perform physical assessment and health education activities, and do them well, then these services must be part of the contract in what is expected to be provided by nurses.

Two areas of concern in community nursing practice have been identified: the unclear accountability (to individuals, communities or physicians?) which thereby confuses clients' expectations of what they will receive from nurses, and lack of reimbursement for autonomous practice. In effect, public health nurses, who have been sanctioned legally as professional, rarely have had the authority or access to practice that way, even though actual service given often is professional.

Nurses, being the creative and political beings that they are, have managed to enrich paid services with free and rarely expected professional ones. With other health care workers legally laying claim to services provided as extra by public health nurses, it is imperative that the latter's contracts now include physical assessment, initiation of nursing therapy based on nursing diagnosis, and health education. These should be required and legitimate nursing services.

Physical assessment is merely a technique used by many health care workers. How the findings are used is what determines one kind of practice. In other words, it is perfectly legitimate for physiotherapists to use data as a basis for range of motion exercises and it is appropriate for physician's assistants to use physical assessment to provide M.D.s with data about possible disease. It is appropriate for nurses to use physical assessment to identify potential or real health deficits and prescribe appropriate therapy, and to identify pathological changes from normal that would be referred to M.D.s. What is not appropriate is for the generic physical assessment skill to be used by someone to provide therapy that belongs to another profession.

PUBLIC HEALTH NURSE AS COMMUNITY NURSE

Public health nursing has the historical role of providing medically directed convalescent care in the home and some screening and care in clinics. These are the two primary kinds of care for which such nurses are paid. To provide true community nursing, the title, the contract, and the care delivery must change.

Nurses in public health agencies are responding to the same professional challenges as those in any setting: initiation of problem-oriented charting to demonstrate the use and effectiveness of nursing diagnosis, use of available data to identify real and potential health deficits, and learning and using the full complement of physical assessment skills. These activities still are available generally in the community only to those receiving reimbursed home medical care or those visiting the clinics for specially advertised services. Unfortunately, the assessment and diagnosis skills still are extra. The time needed to develop and provide these services has not been built into the existing busy schedule of reimbursable care.

New expectations, new changes, and new delivery systems must be developed. The public has come to expect professional nursing in the community, and yet the service is expendable and in jeopardy because it is not required or reimbursed. Employers and third party payers are not looking for or paying for the professional nursing services. Important, necessary, and cost-effective medical assistance and specific disease detection are being offered under the guise of public health nursing. Important and valuable professional nursing care also is developing concurrently as a result of these nurses' having medical access to convalescent or special clinic clients. What needs to change is the equation between extra and necessary nursing care. If community nurses are working as nurses they must give nursing care. That is not to say that existing medical care should not be part of that package. Nurses certainly can do both, unlike physician's assistants who can perform only medical assistance. But nursing contracts and expectations of employers must reflect the professional practice written in state nurse practice acts, and must require professional nursing service when the job incumbent and title are nurse.

Reimbursement for professional nursing services must be accomplished before any contract, written or verbal, between nurse and client or nurse and employer can be accepted. If an employer or client now can receive reimbursement from third party payers for nursing care only when ordered by physicians, what kind of altruism or moral feeling could be expected to induce them to opt for out-of-pocket or unreimbursed nurse-directed services instead? Third party payers need to be shown evidence that the cost of providing professional nursing is less than the cost of the effects on people's health from not receiving it. Reimbursable nursing care in the community may be mostly identification and treatment of individuals at risk for medical problems and of those experiencing or at risk of other health problems open to nursing resolution.

Without those services, those persons sooner or later may end up in a very expensive and unpleasant medical or social crisis. Preventive nursing care can decrease the occurrence and resulting costs of some of these crises in the community. Results to be stressed in obtaining third party reimbursement for professional nursing services might include:

- decreased percent of hospital readmissions for sufferers of a chronic disease such as diabetes
- lower absenteeism in school/industry where health counseling and individual care contracts are developed
- fewer known hypertensives in crisis when provided with exercise, diet, and other health counseling and monitoring

The measurement of each of these factors should be carried out at a specified time (two years) after the baseline statistics (without reimbursable nursing care available) have been taken. If third party payers now are paying for the often disastrous effects of a lack of preventive care, it may be an attractive idea financially to fund such a project. The other, even more important, helpful results of such a program are that the individuals served are healthier, happier, and more productive. After all, even if all health and illness care were really free, would not individuals still rather be healthy? Nursing service has been so elusive and difficult to analyze that clients rarely will know when they are missing that service. Nurses, who do know, must honor clients by accepting the title only when the content is there.

All of these arguments could be used for the typical staff nurse in most hospital settings as well. Again, being an employee limits one's abilities to decide the scope of activity. Working in a medical care setting increases the chance that one will provide medical care.

More and more nurses are demanding permanent client assignments, with time to use and document the nursing process as requirements for professional practice. This primary nurse system provides for professional activity. Another problem in hospitals is that nurse can mean L.P.N.s and R.N.s with or without the first professional degree. At least in the community setting, the public health nurse almost always is a professionally educated nurse with a baccalaureate degree.

NEW TITLE, NEW CONTRACT, NEW SERVICE

Nursing in the community must change. Economics demands it, growing professionalism demands it, plans for national health coverage demand it, consumer sophistication and expectation demand it, legal systems demand it. Most of all, the survival of professional nursing care for people demands it. Economically, when highly qualified nurses give only dependent medical care, it is a waste of money. If time, gasoline, planning, and documentation go into a home visit for convalescent medical care only, the taxpayers' money is not being used wisely. The professional making such a visit must broaden the scope and be involved in economically feasible activities such as prevention and identification of health risks. The growing professionalism of nurses and their awareness of legal requirements and evaluation of their practice pose strong reasons for change in the delivery of community nursing service. Consumers are more informed than ever about the quality and completeness of care. Many already are aware of the deficiency in primary care services that will become painfully apparent in any national form of health care. With so many new health workers on the scene, each polishing and marketing a fragment of care that is part of nursing (physician's assistants, health educators), the profession cannot survive without similar marketing and demand for recognition of its services in licensure, certification, contracts, and reimbursement.

The new community nurses also have a primary care focus and clientele. Their services will include the same physical assessment and nursing diagnosis as P.H.N.s, but the contract for care will include expectation and accountability for these as well as for the dependent medical services. The change in title is necessary so that everyone involved—nurse, client, physician, and employer—all know that a new nurse is on the scene with new skills, expectations, and service. Community nurse says something broader than public health nurse.

'YOU CAN'T HAVE ONE WITHOUT THE OTHER'

The change in contract means many things. First, and most concretely, it means that public health agency contracts (big, public funded, and bureaucratic as they usually are) must change to allow time for professional nursing activities. A nurse practitioner friend of mine was offered a job working on a research project on a large federally funded program studying relationships of blood lipids and cardiovascular disease. The physician project director wanted a nurse practitioner because of the regular physical assessments required for participants in the study. He and the nurse practitioner had an argument over the nurse practitioner job description. It went something like this:

M.D.: I will make up the job description since I know the job that needs to be done.

N.P.: You certainly have the prerogative of listing tasks you want accomplished, but I know better than you what an N.P. does.

M.D.: I need you for certain activities and the full scope of N.P. work is irrelevant.

N.P.: I learned techniques so that I could enrich my nursing care. You can't have one without the other. When I am practicing, I am practicing as an N.P., not a technician.

M.D.: But I would be liable for the medical care you want to provide.

N.P.: I would only give care that I am legally certified to give. In that capacity you cannot have liability for my acts as a professional.

The outcome? The two wrote the job description together and it included all the required special duties of the project as well as the access and process of generic nurse practitioner practice. How does this relate to new community nurse contracts? It may not be legitimate to work as a public health nurse and provide only technical, medically dependent services. ("You can't have one without the other.") If community nurses were contracted for dependent care only, all economic feasibility proposals would require that there be enough of those tasks to fill the nurse's working day completely. Obviously this means that professional nursing needs that were identified could not be addressed or resolved. If a nurse is liable for acting on health needs of clients (nurse practice acts, and definition of nursing) negligence could well be claimed in the absence of such care. This notion troubled us when we first began to look at the liability issue inherent in the adoption of nursing diagnosis in state nursing practice acts, and we learned the following:

1. Not every client has unhealthful responses, therefore nurses need not write them or develop them for every one.
2. Those clients who do have unhealthful responses amenable to nursing therapy should have a nurse available and capable of identifying and resolving them.
3. Nurses who fail to identify or act on nursing diagnosis in their clients probably are negligent in the professional practice of nursing.

It is clear, however, that if there is an unhealthful response, the nurse is indeed liable for identifying it, acting on it, and evaluating the effectiveness of those actions. Most if not all public health nurses are providing knowledgeable and valuable professional nursing care, but too often those services are considered peripheral and are fit in around the required tasks. As health problem resolution becomes more identifiable, valuable, and distinct from medicine, clients will be looking for that service. If nurses are busy with other things, some new professional will appear, unfettered by other demands and be hired as the health educator, the counselor, the assessor of health status. It will be too late to exclaim, "I do that too." Nurses should demand time and money now for the priority practice of their professional service. This evolves by developing appropriate contracts in the public health agencies, hospitals, and ambulatory care settings. The other kind of contract is the one between nurse and client.

NURSE CONTRACTS WITH CLIENTS

Measurable accountability and success depend on a clear, objective outcome. Although one can be accountable for process alone (e.g., the nurse carries out certain assessment and therapy), the final accountability is based on:

1. concurrence between client and therapist about what the goals are
2. successful achievement of those goals or thorough evaluation of intervening factors that compromised achievement

Any contract between a client and the community nurse implies responsibilities, accountability, and liability for both. Responsibilities have to do with input, activities, and commitment. The client is responsible for identifying areas of health concern and for helping to develop and carry out a plan to protect that person's health. The nurse is responsible for more definitive problem identification, including interpretation of signs and symptoms of health problems that the lay person may not detect. For instance, laboratory reports may indicate anemia, allergy, chronic infection, or hypertension and its beginning sequelae, or the meaning behind insidious changes in effect, or the presence of masses, enlarged organs, or lymphadenopathy. Identifying the presence of these findings is the responsibility of a nurse offering primary health care.

Both client and nurse also have accountability to one another in such a contract, the nurse ultimately for identifying and carrying out therapy that alleviates a health problem, and the client for doing all that individual can by carrying out prescribed therapy to meet the health goals. Compliance with mutually agreed upon therapy is the essential ingredient in client accountability.

Liability is the professional's jeopardy for not doing the job inherent in the legal practice of nursing and in the client contract for not performing as agreed. Liability in nursing is just beginning to be defined. The reason for this is that nursing, as a dependent practice of medicine, was liable only for doing or not doing medically ordered work. When one is only part of a process being directed by someone else, liability is limited to actions inappropriately carried out (wrong order or improper performance or omission). The nurse then is liable for a negative outcome, but only on the basis of actions ordered or put into an institutional protocol. Until now, nurses rarely have been liable for omission or negligence in performing activities identified and directed by nurses for health therapy. That kind of liability is growing in direct response to how well nurses are fulfilling their autonomous functions.

The case of *Darling v. Charleston Community Memorial Hospital* resulted in a landmark decision for nurse and institutional liability.[1] In this situation, a boy, hospitalized with a leg injury, eventually had his leg amputated as a result of negligent care. The physician did not heed repeated concerns voiced by the nurses regarding the tightness of the leg cast and the circulatory status of the boy's leg. The nurses did not carry their concerns to any authority other than the physician. The far reaching implications of that landmark case decision include the finding that ultimate responsibility for care rests with the board of trustees, and individual responsibility is present for all care-givers and their superiors to move complaints and concerns upward in the administrative hierarchy until appropriate action is taken. As nursing becomes recognized as an independent practice, so will this liability for outcomes grow.

Clients incur liability for not carrying out actions toward improved health outcome or for not giving full data concerning problem identification. I know of two instances where physicians have denied their continued services to clients who persist in smoking. They have made it clear that medical therapy is to no avail and a waste of the physician's time if the client refuses to act as instructed. The client therefore is liable for cessation of professional services if the person does not comply with healthful behavior or fails to provide complete data.

HEALTH ACHIEVEMENTS AT RISK

Much of the success in reaching health goals depends on activities farther afield than those involving only the community nurse and the client. The two do not function in a vacuum. The nurse needs to direct health therapy in such an individual way that the risks inherent in other client activities are covered. It is not always appropriate to say to the client, "do as I say or find yourself another nurse." Here are some examples of flexible (realistic) practice that allows for individual life styles that are not optimally healthy and yet do not put the nurse in jeopardy for not achieving certain health goals.

The Case of Sara the Arthritic

An elderly woman we shall call Sara has had rheumatoid arthritis for nearly 60 years. During that time the exacerbations and contractures have been treated in a variety of ways, including partial bone removal in her feet and, more recently, weekly gold injections as maintenance therapy. Sara feels well and has great trust in her rheumatologist. She came to our clinic to register for primary care coverage. She is not taking aspirin for joint pain ("my neighbor told me it would make my stomach bleed") and relies entirely on the gold therapy. On consultation, we learned that her rheumatologist planned to continue gold therapy, giving her injections weekly and relying on the primary care clinic to monitor and care for her other health needs. Gold is a potential nephrotoxin, especially so in the aged or in people like Sara who have a low tolerance for drinking a great deal of fluids.

Although our own nonspecialist thoughts questioned long-term gold therapy between flare-ups, the research in recent literature verified such therapy, although the potential kidney damage is very much of a health risk for Sara. We were able to devise a plan with Sara that allowed continued compliance with her rheumatologist's therapy and with our idea of adequate compliant primary health care. We decided to obtain frequent and regular urinalysis testing (monthly at the time of one of her weekly gold injection treatments), alerted her to any warning signs and symptoms such as flank pain, lessened or no output of urine, and asked her to try a regime of increased water intake during the days she was home. In this way we covered the risks of other therapy in ways that were acceptable in our overall accountability for Sara's health.

The Case of Kim and the Pill

Another example of managing health risk is Kim, a young mother on birth control pills. Kim is a single working woman, age 26, with a two-year-old daughter and a history of one elective abortion, moderate smoking, and varicose veins in both legs. Her gynecologist continues BCPs as contraceptive of choice (an earlier IUD had caused too many subjective complaints from Kim). On consultation, he shared with us his reasons. Kim was young, thin, and active and therefore did not pose the risks for emboli that some women do. She is sexually active and requires effective birth control. The gynecologist sees her every six months for an examination and prescription renewal.

Kim came to us for her annual physical examination and for primary care services for herself and her daughter. We were concerned with the health risks involved in BCPs and and spent much time trying to convince Kim either to give up smoking or try another form of birth control. We learned that the IUD experience had occurred a few years before her daughter's birth and therefore a retrial now might prove far more satisfactory. Kim wanted to think about a change, especially after hearing the statistics involving smokers and BCPs. She knew that the choice was hers to make, but that her responsibility in opting for BCPs would be regular examinations and blood work with us so the effects of the risk could be monitored.

In community nursing as in all other areas of the profession, clients and nurses decide on the outcome and both then become accountable. With Kim, the primary outcome desired was effective birth control. For this, certain risks (for Kim) and monitoring (for the nurse) were assumed. Our contract for care included extra visits and costs for Kim if BCPs were her choice, or fewer visits and tests if the IUD were chosen.

The Case of Barbara the Vegetarian

Sometimes the conflict in health risks is not other medical therapy but simply the chosen life style of the client. Once again, the contract for care will involve common goals with separate responsibilities. Barbara is a primary care client who is a strict vegetarian. She supplements her diet with high daily doses of vitamins and minerals. Some of the amounts are excessive (50,000 units of Vitamin A) and none of her diets includes a combination of foods to provide complete proteins. Barbara is a Jehovah's Witness and a few years earlier had refused postoperative blood transfusions even though her hemoglobin was extremely low. Her current iron intake (and supplement) were maintaining her hemoglobin at an acceptable level. However, we were worried about high Vitamin A dosage, calcium crystals in her urine, and her complaint in the clinic that "I feel run down and always seem to have a cold."

The apparent deficiency in protein could contribute to increased susceptibility to virus infections and decreased energy. We addressed the nutrition issue with her, including the risk of liver damage from excessive Vitamin A and the possibility that urinary calcium could be a result of the high oral doses of calcium. Barbara was resistant to change the vitamin and mineral regime. She had recovered from a very serious illness (cancer) five years before and fully believed her diet and supplements were responsible. We were able, however, to devise food combinations that she liked and could afford and that provided complete protein. With continuing information regarding Vitamin A, its storage, and its natural sources, Barbara may yet come to accept decreased intake, and the same may happen for her calcium intake. Meanwhile, our contract for care includes an agreement that she knowingly accepts the risk of liver damage and kidney stones from her self-medication. She has been advised of the effects and their symptoms and carries that liability herself.

The Case of Howard the Heavy

Howard is a middle-aged man, overweight, hypertensive, compulsive, and independent. He works part time and does the cooking and housework for his invalid wife. He has gone on weight-reducing diets prescribed in our clinic many times. He loses the weight, returns to his former habits, the weight goes back on, and the blood pressure goes back up. He seemed as frustrated as we were to find, at his regular hypertension management visit, that he again had reached a blood pressure and a weight far above acceptable. The physician in our group sat down with a sigh, tossed the chart on the chair between them, and said, "OK, Howard, what now? More of the same? Another see-saw on the scale?"

Howard had his own idea, his own diet, and his own schedule. His contract with us was four pounds' weight loss a month and we would help him do it his way. His way essentially was to decrease calories, but included ice cream once in a while, a sweet roll on Sunday, and perhaps some gravy on mashed potatoes. We worked with him to be sure the potatoes were not a substitute for vegetables, or the sweet roll for fruit. His responsibility to us was (1) weight loss as listed: four to six pounds per month and (2) if the blood pressure stayed up even with the weight loss, he would comply with a stricter regime we would prescribe. Our responsibility in the contract was: (1) regular weight and blood pressure monitoring, (2) diet instruction as needed, and (3) assessment and action on inadequate risk resolution.

How easy it is to do these things and how commonsensical it all is. And yet, to devise such a contract is to do many things:

1. It spells out expectations and responsibilities.
2. It makes a team of client and nurse for common goals.
3. It spells out risks and accomplishments.
4. It is motivating to both.

A client-nurse contract is most useful and most possible in ambulatory or community nursing. In these settings the client has the opportunity to choose health goals and to act on them. The definition of nursing as being potentiation of optimum health is very much reflected in the concept of a health contract.

PRIORITIES AND LIABILITIES

Priorities among goals and failure of goal achievement with its attendant liability are part of contract development. A person may have a number of real or at-risk health problems. Improper nutrition, obesity, smoking, or lack of exercise all may be present, may be amenable to some common therapies, and yet may seem overwhelming if addressed together. Perhaps obesity and improper nutrition will be controlled best (at least initially) if the client does not forego smoking at the same time; perhaps exercise and smoking can be addressed together while the person still enjoys ice cream and mashed potatoes with gravy. The nurse may have professionally determined priorities that say one or the other set of circumstances should be worked on first, but two effective results ensue if the client decides priorities:

1. Choice tends to promote commitment.
2. Commitment tends to promote success, and success promotes further commitment.

There are times when risks are so varied that clients must be encouraged to follow professional direction. For instance, with an overweight smoker with EKG changes and angina suggesting serious cardiac ischemia, smoking must outrank weight reduction as a priority goal. Sometimes, too, there is an umbrella goal—one that will cover others. For instance, proper nutrition also may resolve obesity, or helping a client better handle anxiety may reduce smoking and hypertension. Therefore, client preference is motivating and to be encouraged, except in choices that may affect life or when a directed choice will include the self-identified one. In any professional service, a desired outcome that justifies professional therapy and client compliance is identified. A measurable and client-valued outcome helps make the whole process of care understandable and acceptable to the person and gives both that individual and the nurse a sense of accomplishment together when achieved.

The idea of failure of goal achievement raises questions:

1. Who is liable, client or nurse?
2. Why was success not achieved?
3. Was the goal possible or reasonable? Were there intervening factors?
4. Was the therapy appropriate for the goal desired?

Many of these questions are new to the evaluation of autonomous nursing care, whose records have not included regular assessment about what those actions achieved. Most often the nursing activities were linked in some standardized way to the alleviation of a medical problem. Rarely were they aimed at client-chosen health status improvement. Although nurses learn by trial and error and by apprenticing with an experienced nurse what works for clients, rational approaches to an outcome based on given regimes have been rare. There is no sure answer as to what approaches work best in given circumstances. What about obesity? Is there a right way to resolve it? Certainly Howard's way is not tried universally, and yet for compulsive, overweight, and hypertensive men his way may be the method of choice for weight reduction.

This problem of lack of research about what nursing therapies work best is the one most likely to cause failure in goal achievement. There was a time when the medical profession did not have a predictable outcome for a given therapy and it used a variety of approaches to treat such problems as heart attacks (strict long-term bed rest, restricted activity thereafter, or short-term inactivity only and dietary fat reduction). Now there is far more consensus on proper therapy because of research on both methods. Nursing needs to develop its own research on what is most appropriate for treating given health problems. As that develops, liability will be clearer.

Professionals are liable for prescribing the care with the greatest likelihood of success. No professional would accept liability for actual success in any individual situation. The federally legislated professional evaluation of care system (PSRO) is being developed so that physicians agree on certain desired and expected results of care based on medical diagnosis. For instance, every person having an appendectomy is expected to survive, be discharged in ambulatory condition without permanent disability, fever, or drainage within a few days. There are exceptions for those previously disabled or with intervening health problems not directly associated with the procedure (stroke, preexisting pneumonia, etc.). When the desired outcome is not achieved, the process is examined. Standards for adequate procedure also are developed so that physicians are liable for inadequate or inappropriate therapy when the desired outcome is not achieved.

Neither the nurse nor the physician, however, can be accountable for success; they can be responsible only for proper diagnosis and for following the therapy with the greatest chance of success. The therapy most likely to succeed and a well-thought-out diagnosis are joined by a third criterion, which together make success most likely. That criterion is to accept only clients one can help legitimately. In primary care settings, the burden falls on professionals to refer cases to appropriate other experts when they do not have all the skills or all the knowledge to do the whole job needed.

In a community health setting, nursing is aimed at convalescence, screening, promotion, and prevention. Clients with the needs best met by nursing in this setting are:

1. those receiving home visits for convalescent care who may be looking at health as a priority in their life because of a recent but now resolved illness
2. those seen in their home environment, which helps the nurse identify problems in health achievements (crowding, poor nutrition, noise, pollution, many stairs to climb, etc.)
3. those who visit health assessment or screening clinics who have self-identified themselves as open to health improvement and usually are not ill at the time

Health assessment and therapy provided by the community nurse to individuals is the core of primary care nursing. It occurs wherever there is professional nursing. The assessment, therapy, and maximization of health that occur in community nursing are just as beneficial and important to individuals there as in any other setting, but the main focus and accountability is improved health levels for the community as a whole. How this comes about without compromising individual care can be demonstrated in two ways: (1) by addressing different care priorities in individual clients and (2) by developing a nursing process diagram for community nursing practice.

COMMUNITY PRIORITIES BECOME INDIVIDUAL THERAPY

When individuals are treated by nurses for real or potential health problems there usually are a number of ways to identify and assign priorities to those problems. For example, any client may have many at-risk physical behaviors such as smoking, poor nutrition, overeating, alcohol abuse, or inadequate exercise, and also may have environmental health risk factors at work (toxins, noise, machinery) or home (crowding, pollution, disease, rats, poor lighting, rickety stairs). Such assessments also include attitudinal and coping factors such as anxiety, grief, anger, or depression that influence health. Clearly, any number of clients may demonstrate more than one or two of these problems. Resolution of some may require solving other problems first or concurrently. Sometimes problems will disappear without specific therapy if an overall umbrella problem is solved first.

The nurse is accountable to the community for having a broader vision than individual problem solving so that priorities of care for individuals are decided by identifying priority community problems. If a community has a particularly broad-based air pollution problem, then (barring other serious individual problems), respiratory care such as screening, prevention, and health promotion would be a priority for the community nurse and clients. If there were an inordinate number of heart attacks or acquired heart disease in the community, then priority for detection and treatment with individual clients would be carried out in the areas of diet prescription, stress testing and exercise, antismoking campaigns, etc.

Most primary clients of nurses are either without overt disease or symptoms or have attained a stable condition with a chronic disease. Because of this they are more likely to have a number of noncritical health problems. Each individual would receive care for health problems on a priority basis determined by the community-wide concern or occurrence. If there were a widespread need for stress testing and exercise, and it were one of the client's needs but not necessarily that individual's first priority, it still would be provided before other therapy because of the community's priority. If, however, an individual had one problem clearly more serious than others, it would be treated before the No. 1 community concern. This kind of approach may seem both simplistic and unrealistic. And yet, if the scope and method of community nursing practice is examined closely, it makes more sense.

Every profession has a practice component to improve individual welfare. Community-based and community-accountable professionals such as public defenders, public health nurses and physicians, and public school teachers have a primary accountability to a community. Although care is provided for individuals, it is the improved community welfare that is required. For instance, the school teacher who provides knowledge and motivation to the student most in need of those services at the expense of the rest of the class has not done the required job. The same is true for the public defender who ignores individuals with lesser needs for legal defense so that he can best serve the client with greatest risk. This is not legitimate practice for one with community responsibility. The analogy is the same for the community nurse.

Individuals of varying need seek nursing care for real or potential health problems. Those common health problems that when treated will benefit the most people are the priority for the community nurse. Although nursing care still is provided to individuals, the methods of assessment and treatment also include groups. Assessment clinics can be focused solely on respiratory insufficiency or hypertension identification or other discrete problems. Treatment can be given in groups, and sometimes is even more effective that way (quit-smoking groups, for example).

NURSING PROCESS FOR COMMUNITY OUTCOMES

The process applied by community health nurses has individual and community participants and measurements to evaluate effectiveness for both types. Following is an outline for such a process.

Step 1: Data

> A. community trends: hospital admissions, absenteeism causes, episodic visits
> B. health assessment of individuals

Step 2: Diagnosis

> A. interpretation of data regarding unhealthful responses and etiology for both communities and individuals
> B. priority listing of diagnosis depending on:
> 1. how widespread the problems are
> 2. the feasibility of successful intervention (resources and client/community motivation)
> 3. the time and money available

4. whether appropriate for nursing intervention rather than referral

Step 3: Goals

A. outcome: broad measurements agreed on by community
B. individual health measurements
These two may differ in that community measures may be final (reduced numbers of heart attacks) whereas individual measures may
be different for different persons (reduced blood pressure, lowered
serum lipids, or weight loss that had put them at risk for a heart
attack).

Step 4: Planning

A. agreement on therapeutic activities with community participants,
both providers and recipients.
B. priorities for care and identification of resources, payment, and
referrals

Step 5: Implementation

A. community group intervention to increase motivation and knowledge for behavioral changes
B. individual sessions for hands-on care and monitoring

Step 6: Evaluation

A. community goals reached
B. individual goals achieved
C. correlation between the two
D. interpretation and analysis of findings, including health level
(individual or community), cost and community satisfaction
Sometimes the goal can be reached but the resulting trade-offs are
unacceptable. If the pollution and respiratory dysfunction were decreased 10 percent with a resulting 50 percent increase in unemployment from industry shutdown, the community might not be
satisfied with the outcome.

This nursing process outlines activities for community health problem
diagnosis, treatment, and resolution. This is done by identifying trends,
resources, and motivation for treatment, and trade-offs in accomplishment.
The treatment may be activities without specific client contact—changing

pollution control devices, improving structural deficits in housing, or obtaining wider eligibility for food stamps. These are uniquely community interventions. Or the treatment may be the same individual contacts as in ambulatory or institutional settings such as respiratory testing and exercises, nutrition counseling, or skin care. Community nurses are accountable for improved health levels of their community through both public health advocacy programs and individual treatment.

As public health advocates (e.g., pollution control, housing improvement, food stamps), nonnurse public health professionals can provide the treatment. Therefore, the reasons for including these services in community nurse practice are important. First, the health problems that are caused by pollution, inadequate nutrition, and poor housing are best and earliest detected by a nurse. These are nursing diagnoses. Second, individual treatment may be needed for resolution, as well as the community-based improvements (respiratory testing as well as pollution control; diet counseling and laboratory studies as well as food stamps), and these are part of nursing therapy.

Specialists with public health training such as epidemiologists, environmental scientists, and toxicologists can identify causes of illness or imperiled health. However, they do not have a therapeutic practice that covers individual identification or treatment. Community nurses do and have the specific public health perspective to identify etiology while treating individuals. Individual findings may suggest trends in community-wide health problems and broad community intervention as well as individual treatment. During the evaluation phase, the individual and the community both remain important and must be monitored for the comprehensive evaluation. Again, only a nurse can do both. Community health is assessed, treated, and improved through both individual and community therapy.

The community nursing process outline helps demonstrate the interaction of individual and community as joint participants in health achievement and evaluation. It also points up again the conflicts between goals that may increase the health of some individuals (respiratory problems) while at the same time, through unemployment, put the health of others more at risk. This is a decision a community must make. The nurse can assist by clarifying risk potential, therapeutic cost, and alternatives. For instance, industrial air pollution can go down and unemployment stay the same if the industrial community agrees to provide an expensive pollution control system with monies previously planned for improved pensions, more vacations, or aesthetic changes. There are many kinds of human welfare, and health professionals often do not understand why the public will not always opt for the health benefit over others. The reality is that communities will not always do that, and it is the community prerogative to make those choices.

PAYERS ARE NOT ALWAYS BENEFICIARIES

The community nurse's role in such decisions is to paint a clear and complete picture of the effects of neglected health on the community as well as an honest and knowledgeable sketch of costs to the community for the preventive care. One main difference in this equation applied to the community is that those paying for care or preventive services are not necessarily the recipient of the benefits. That always has been true in public-financed ventures and accounts in part for low motivation in compliance.

Community nurses identify community health problems and trends. Infections, disease, nutritional deficits or excesses, environmental pollutants and hazards, smoking, and exercise deficits are some of the health issues that community nurses can assess by presenting effects on individual health status. Case-finding efforts include screening clinics for specific findings, health history and physical examinations, and reviews of most common causes of hospitalization and industrial absences. From analysis of these findings, the health problems most prevalent or at risk in the community are identified. Individuals with identified health problems are treated or referred for care and the most common problems are addressed in followups that are within the scope of community nursing, such as screening to determine whether unidentified other persons may have symptoms or disease, and health education and group counseling.

Community nurses are committed to raising community health standards and levels. To do so means interaction with individuals after community assessments are made to identify those with the most common problems and risks. Community benefits are not always desired by individuals; what groups define as good is not always acceptable to individuals. Communities want to know their fish markets will not sell contaminated clams and yet individuals want to preserve their freedom to collect and eat clams without interference. Communities agree that hypertension screening is a valuable way to use public funds but individuals identified as hypertensive may resist medication and diet therapy. Communities may agree that industry should be under sanctions for air pollution and yet individuals will not refrain from smoking, or leaf burning, or excessive automobile use.

Translating community health goals into individual health behavior is difficult, yet higher community health goals require changes in health behavior at the individual level. Community nurses often can gain access to individual testing and community health data (school absences, hospital admission diagnoses, etc.) to determine priorities for health intervention, but successful intervention requires changes in individual behavior. Individual access for this kind of therapy often is denied or apathetic and yet the community nurse is accountable for helping clients adopt community health standards and desires as individual goals. Altruism probably will not work. Societal responsibility can be motivating, especially if there are individual penalties. One proposal is that clients who comply to achieve community health goals (e.g., not smoking to lower the incidence of respiratory dysfunction) will have free care (community tax monies, perhaps) for respiratory illness. Those who do not comply are not so insured. This kind of sanction makes much more sense when a national plan for health care is adopted that not only helps finance care for everyone but also provides differences in access to care based on individual self-care compliance (e.g., nonsmokers have first priority for scarce resources for respiratory care).

Penalties are not the only factors that work. Positive achievements that benefit both the individual and the community are the easiest to promote. When there are conflicts, they usually occur because individuals are not getting enough return on their investments. This is where there is a need for more precise information or future effects based on the current investment of money, and on adoption of difficult new health behaviors. Payoffs on health practices are not yet known well enough to be motivating factors and, even when known, the time is so long between investment and payoff that people are not motivated.

COMPLEXITY AND CHALLENGE IN THE COMMUNITY

Community nurses require the consensus of a defined community to act on health achievements. The professional ability to recognize goals with the greatest investment potential means that strong input is required from nurses when communities make decisions. The collaboration and contract between a community and the nurse make possible highly productive achievements.

The physician members required in any optimal health system fit into the community system the same way they do in any nurse-client-physician triad: to make definitive medical diagnoses, treat individuals, and assist in calculating cost, method, and effectiveness of disease resolution. The nurse-physician collaboration is essential here, as elsewhere, to assure that both disease resolution and preventive/promotive care are provided.

The greater complexity in this system arises in the community setting because goals there depend on individual behavior and because of the whole range of causes for which there is no purely nursing resolution or medical cure. Poor lighting, unsanitary conditions, noise and air pollution, and inadequate money for food, shelter, and clothing all are health problems that depend on intervention other than health therapy for solution. Community nurses and physicians therefore need the public health perspectives of group risk and need and the special knowledge of epidemiology, environmental health, group process, and political and ethical management as well as the generic requirements of their unique professional practice in order to be effective.

NOTE

1. *Nursing and the Law* (Germantown, Md.: Aspen Systems Corp., 1975), pp. 8-9.

RECOMMENDED READING

Freeman, Ruth B., *Community Health Nursing Practice*. Philadelphia: W. B. Saunders Co., 1970.

Focus on Health Maintenance and Prevention of Illness. Wakefield, Mass.: Contemporary Publishing Co., 1975.

Chapter 7

Autonomous Practice: The Vision and the Reality

*"Like one that stands upon a promontory,
And spies a far-off shore where he would tread,
Wishing his foot were equal with his eye."*
Shakespeare, in *King Henry VI*, Part III.

There is an old saw in publishing that says events occur in the real world in inverse proportion to how frequently they appear in print. It seems that the idea of autonomous nursing practice is filling the books and journals, yet those of us actually working with nurses and clients are experiencing a surge in professional practice everywhere. The thoughts and passions in these pages reflect what is happening already, and the message here is to enlarge and strengthen that endeavor so that more nurses will develop autonomous practice for their clients.

As that development goes forward, nurses must believe that they can make their vision of professional care a reality. It will take creativity, commitment, knowledge, skill, wiles, and strategies, but it will happen. The barriers are there: the entrenched and smug status quo beneficiaries, the economic questions of long-term measurement of here-and-now investment, and the soft, amorphous, and valuable element called nursing, which has been so hard to define and separate from other professions.

Three thoughts on the nature of nursing may help strengthen the direction this important development is taking:

1. Nurses know better than anyone else when nursing care is needed.
2. Nursing, as with all professions, will continue to grow in knowledge and skill to meet the changing needs of people.
3. Nurses are autonomous but do not work in isolation; rather they function as unique professionals who give their richest service in

collaboration with others: physicians, clients (both individual and community) and other nonhealth-related professionals.

Because nurses know best when nursing is needed, they must have access to detect health problems, have authority to direct actions for problem resolution, and have accountability for the outcome. This kind of system includes direct reimbursement and acknowledgment by purchasers of care that professional nursing is what they are buying. Primary access to clients is essential, but there is a need to go even farther. People need to learn to identify signs and symptoms that demonstrate their own need for nursing care. Also needed is an enormous public effort to educate everyone about what health achievements are possible through nursing therapy and how to identify behavior or environment that may pose risks for optimal health. The thrust for primary care skills (complete data gathering skills, as well as diagnostic and management competency) must encompass all nurses, regardless of the setting, since assessment and management of professional nursing care takes place in all settings.

THE GROWTH IS NATURAL, NOT EXPANDED OR NEW

Because all professions grow in knowledge and skill to meet changing needs, there is no reason to label this natural growth in nursing the expanded role or the new nurse. All professions are flexible. Only technicians are limited to tasks or process boundaries. Where nurses or other professionals have specialized knowledge or skill in their profession, the title and authority should be clear. For instance, pediatric nurse practitioners specialize in assessment and primary care of children, but their generic ability to follow the nursing process is the same as with a geriatric nurse practitioner.

Should all nurses be nurse practitioners? To the extent that nurse practitioner means the ability to obtain and act on primary data, yes. Nurses everywhere should know how to obtain and interpret the comprehensive information needed to provide care. Even though most nurse practitioners are trained for primary care, the same assessment and management skills are needed in nonprimary settings (hospitals, rehabilitation centers, day hospitals, and hospices). Nurse practitioner probably is a title that will eventually describe all professional nurses, for the practitioner skills should belong to all professional nurses regardless of where they care for people.

Because nursing is a unique service, as are all professions, it must be acknowledged as having the access, authority, and accountability for that service. However, autonomous practice does not mean practice in isolation. It means having autonomous authority and decision making in nursing situations.

However, people, in their wonderful and frustrating complexity, rarely present a nicely boxed nursing problem. The reality is that people's health needs are mixed up with many other factors, including their family roles, work requirements, life styles, and medical problems. To try to pick out the pieces that are purely nursing and treat them in isolation often is impossible.

COLLABORATION A KEY WORD

Autonomy in nursing thrives on collaboration. Therapy is provided separately and together—separate and distinct for nursing diagnostic identification and therapy direction, and together in working on joint plans and results with the client and other involved care-givers. Nursing therapy often is most effective when given in concert with care provided by other professionals. Unhealthful responses can be caused or influenced by medical, sociological, economic, environmental, and political factors. Nurses cannot be expert in all of these areas, and indeed should not be. However, identification of the unhealthful response (nursing diagnosis) and intervention to erase or alleviate the causal factors often can be done through group or team efforts. Air pollution, for example, is best addressed by doctors, economists, industrialists, environmentalists, and nurses— certainly more effectively than by nurses alone.

Neither the setting nor the legitimate presence of other professionals compromises or limits the delivery of professional nursing services. Many contend that professional nursing has no place in the hospital setting because the client is there for acute medical care. Certainly that is the priority, but if nurses work there, then clients must be recipients of their nursing care, resolving health problems. It may not be the priority, but it must be a component. Even when clients are primarily receiving other professional care, when nurses become part of the matrix of therapy it is never enough simply to fulfill the dependent tasks of another's direction. It is insufficient to give one (dependent care) without the other (autonomous care). Wherever clients need nursing service, it must be available, assured, and provided by comprehensive, skilled, and qualified professionals.

WHAT OF THE FUTURE?

The future for autonomous nursing depends on client awareness and demand for the services and on the continued development and identification of nurses fully able to provide them. Nurses who are true professionals in the sense of knowledge, skill, commitment, and accountability are compromised in the public view because so many lesser qualified persons also lay claim to the title "nurse." "A nurse is a nurse is a nurse" means that there is a guarantee for only the lowest common denominator of service. Nurse practitioner, nurse clinician, licensed practical nurse, and registered professional nurse all are attempts to be more definitive about who is who, but the only ones who really understand the differences are other nurses. The future of professional nursing will depend in part on effective measures to help clients know who is caring for them.

The other part of developing client awareness and demand for professional services is to define what health problems are solved by nursing therapy and what the signs and symptoms of those health problems are so that clients will know when to refer themselves to nurses. Clients also need to know what kind of health goals are possible through nursing therapy. This is particularly necessary for those who have no actual health problems to be identified but would be appropriate nursing clients for health promotion or preventive care. Such a problem list, with signs and symptoms, is being developed by practicing nurses, educators, and administrators through the National Task Force on Classification of Nursing Diagnosis.[1] An edited version for consumer reference would be valuable.

Even with sufficient highly qualified and skilled professional nurses and concurrent client sophistication about what they can achieve with health therapy, the service will not survive without direct (autonomous) reimbursement. If clients recognize professional nursing service and want it, the mechanisms for reimbursement will follow. Reimbursement will be a natural by-product of providing a high quality measurable and valued service.

If nurses are directing and giving nursing care, then they are the ones to be paid for it. If professional nursing service is not available without direct payment, then clients (the best lobbying force there is) will demand it from their insurance coverage and, when paying out of pocket, will pay nurses for their care. When a national health plan insuring or subsidizing health care is adopted, new federal guidelines will be developed for reimbursement. Nursing can best be ready for that day by developing a measurable list of nursing diagnoses and health outcomes for which it is accountable and for which it should be paid.

THE RISE IN NEW HEALTH PROBLEMS

In years past the greatest opportunities for nursing care were in medical settings. Disease, infection, and trauma were by far the major areas of medical intervention and nursing assistance. Highly technological care was developed and people came to expect, and sometimes to value, the passive sick role where they were treated in dramatic ways and their own responsibilities for cure or prevention were few.[2] Expectations are changing both for health professionals and for their clients.

Health problems now are more those resulting from environmental and occupational causes, life styles that are unhealthy, and the stress and anxiety of modern living. Disease, infection, and trauma still are with us, but they are a much smaller percentage of health problems. Physicians who have always been trained for and practice in pathology and disease resolution, now are expanding for their own survival into areas of treating unhealthful responses and activities that heretofore were thought of as voluntary social behavior (smoking, obesity, inadequate exercise).

If it was poor use of professional nursing to be involved only in dependent medical activities, then what should be thought of if the treatment of unhealthful responses becomes the new turf of medicine, with nursing again as the assistant? It is one thing to be an assistant to a different profession, but quite another to be an assistant within one's own profession. It is quite clear that the whole area of prevention and promotion will be the primary focus of clients, health professionals, and payers of care in the years ahead. It is a legitimate and rich area for professional nursing, but nurses must be ready and recognized as autonomous professionals in every sense of the word in order to take the leadership in health in the future.

This is not a new idea, but it is revolutionary. Single-minded commitment from nursing will be needed to make the vision a reality—to "make the foot equal with the eye." People indeed will be receiving individual care for unhealthful behavior because they are becoming vitally interested in health promotion and prevention. Will nurses be directing and leading those services? It is up to them to articulate their professional claim and their skill and to demonstrate their autonomous excellence.

NOTES

1. Summary of the Third National Conference on Classification of Nursing Diagnoses, St. Louis University School of Nursing, 1978.

2. David Mechanic, "Health and Illness in Technological Societies," *Hastings Center Studies*, 1, no. 3 (1973).

RECOMMENDED READING

Mauksh, Hans O. "Nursing: Churning for a Change?" *Handbook of Medical Sociology*, Englewood Cliffs, N.J.: Prentice-Hall, Inc., 1972.

Kelly, Lucie Young. *Dimensions of Professional Practice*. New York: McMillan Co.

State-by-State Summary of Nurse Practice Acts*

*Adopted from Virginia C. Hall, "Summary of Statutory Provisions Governing Legal Scope of Nursing Practice in the Various States," in *The New Health Professionals,* A. Bliss and E. Cohen, eds. (Germantown, Md.: Aspen Systems Corporation, 1977). Reprinted with permission. ©1977 Aspen Systems Corporation.

If Additional Acts Amendment, Criteria and Conditions Stated

State	Type of Definition	Definition Includes Prohibition Against Acts of Diagnosis and Prescription	Rules and Regulations	Professional Opinion	Education and Training	If New Definition, Incorporated some or all of New York's	Prohibitions of Practice of Medicine in Nurse Practice Act	Exception for Nursing in Medical Practice Act	Physician Supervision of Nurse Practitioners	Degree of Supervision
Alabama	New & Additional Acts Amendment	No	Yes	—	—	Yes	No	No	Required for Nurse Anesthetist	Direct for 30 days, then protocol for midwife
Alaska	Traditional & Additional Acts Amendment	Yes (Applies to "medical" acts only and additional acts not subject to prohibition.)	Yes*	—	—	—	No	No	Collaborative relationship for Nurse-Midwife	
Arizona	Traditional & Additional Acts Amendment[1]	No	Yes*	Yes*	Yes	—	No	Yes (Under physician supervision)	Under direction of and in collaboration with	Presence required for Nurse Anesthetist
Arkansas	Traditional	Yes (Applies to "medical" acts only)	—	—	—	—	No	Yes (Also separate exemption for nurse acting under physician supervision)	Required for Nurse Anesthetist	Presence required
California	New	No	—	—	—	No	No	Yes (For persons lawfully practicing another profession)		As defined by policies and protocols developed for specific setting
Colorado	New & Additional Acts Amendment	No	Yes**	No	Yes	Yes	No	Yes (Also separate exemption for persons acting under physician supervision)	Required	Defined in protocols

	New	No				Yes	Yes	Yes (Under physician supervision)	Not stated
Connecticut		No							
Delaware	Traditional	Yes	–	–	–	–	No	No	Not stated
District of Columbia	No Definition	–	–	–	–	–	No	Yes	Not stated
Florida	Traditional & Additional Acts Amendment	No	Yes	–	–	–	Yes	Yes (Under physician supervision)	Not stated
Georgia	Traditional	No	–	–	–	–	No	Yes (Also separate exemption for persons acting under physician supervision)	Nurse Anesthetists function under direction of physician
Hawaii	Traditional	Yes (Applies to "medical" acts only)	–	–	–	–	No	No (?)²	No specific legislation
Idaho	Traditional & Additional Acts Amendment	Yes	Yes (Applies to "medical" acts only and additional acts not subject to prohibition)	No	–	–	No	No	None referred to but "practice policies" for individuals may so indicate
Illinois	Traditional	Yes (Applies to "medical" acts only)	–	–	–	–	No	Yes (For persons lawfully practicing another profession)	No specific legislation
Indiana	New & Additional Acts Amendment	No	Yes***	No	–	Yes	No	Yes	Required for Nurse Anesthetist
Iowa	New & Additional Acts Amendment	No	–	–	–	Yes	Yes	Yes	No specific regulations
Kansas	Traditional	Yes	–	–	–	–	No	Yes (Also separate exemption for persons acting under physician supervision)	No legislation
Kentucky	Traditional	Yes (Applies to "medical" acts only)	–	–	–	–	No	Yes	No legislation
Louisiana	New & Additional Amendment Act	Yes	Yes	–	–	Yes	No	Yes	Required

If Additional Acts Amendment, Criteria and Conditions Stated

State	Type of Definition	Definition Includes Prohibition Against Acts of Diagnosis and Prescription	Rules and Regulations	Professional Opinion	Education and Training	If New Definition, Incorporated some or all of New York's	Prohibitions of Practice of Medicine in Nurse Practice Act	Exception for Nursing in Medical Practice Act	Physician Supervision of Nurse Practitioners	Degree of Supervision
Maine	Traditional & Additional Acts Amendment	No	No	No	Yes	–	No	No	Physician can delegate certain services	
Maryland	New & Additional Acts Amendment	No	Yes**	Yes*	Yes	Yes	No	Yes (For persons lawfully practicing another profession)	Not stated	
Massachusetts	Traditional & Additional Acts Amendment	No	Yes*	Yes**	Yes	Yes	No	Yes (Applies only to nurses performing "Additional acts")	No regulations	
Michigan	Traditional	Yes (Applies to "medical" acts only)	–	–	–	–	No	Yes (For persons lawfully practicing another profession and separate exemption for persons acting under physician supervision)	No specific legislation	
Minnesota	New	No	–	–	–	Yes	No	Yes (For persons lawfully practicing another profession)	No specific legislation	
Mississippi	Traditional & Additional Acts Amendment	Yes (Applies to "medical" acts only and additional acts not subjected to prohibition)	Yes*	No	No	–	No	No	Not stated	

Missouri	New	No	—	—	Yes	No	Yes	No specific legislation	
Montana	Traditional	Yes	—	—	—	No	Yes	No specific legislation	
Nebraska	New & Additional Amendment Act	Yes, Medicine	Yes	—	Yes	No	Yes (For persons lawfully practicing another profession—not applicable to prescription or administration of drugs)	Required	Specific to each approved expanded role
Nevada	Traditional & Additional Acts Amendment	Yes (Applies to "medical" acts only and additional acts not subject to prohibition)	Yes**	Yes*	—	No	Yes	Collaboration	As agreed in writing
New Hampshire	New & Additional Acts Amendment	Yes (Additional acts not subject to prohibition)	Yes*	Yes**	Yes	No	Yes	Collaboration	Nurse anesthetists function within physical presence of physician
New Jersey	New	No	—	—	Yes	No	Yes (Under physician supervision)	No specific legislation	
New Mexico	Traditional	Yes (Applies to "medical" acts only)	—	—	—	No	Yes (Plus separate exemption for nurse practitioners in certain settings)	Required	
New York	New	No	—	—	Yes	Yes	Yes (For persons lawfully practicing another profession)	No regulations	
North Carolina	Traditional & Additional Acts Amendment	Yes (Applies to "medical" acts only and excepts acts under supervision of physician)	Yes*	No	—	No	Yes (For nursing and those acts "otherwise constituting medical practice" which are permitted by regulations of medical and nursing boards)	Required	Telecommunications, predetermined plan for emergencies, review of practice
North Dakota	Traditional	No	—	—	—	No	No	No regulations	

If Additional Acts Amendment, Criteria and Conditions Stated

State	Type of Definition	Definition Includes Prohibition Against Acts of Diagnosis and Prescription	Rules and Regulations	Professional Opinion	Education and Training	If New Definition, Incorporated some or all of New York's	Prohibitions of Practice of Medicine in Nurse Practice Act	Exception for Nursing in Medical Practice Act	Physician Supervision of Nurse Practitioners	Degree of Supervision
Ohio	Traditional	Yes (Applies to "medical" acts only)	—	—	—	—	Yes	Yes (For nurse anesthetists only, under physician supervision)	Required for nurse-midwife and nurse anesthetist	Nurse anesthetist must work in presence of physician
Oklahoma	Traditional	Yes	—	—	—	—	No	Yes (Under physician supervision)	No regulations	
Oregon	New & Additional Acts Amendment	No	Yes**	Yes*	Yes	Yes	No	Yes	Collaboration	
Pennsylvania	New & Additional Acts Amendment	Yes (Applies to "medical" acts only and additional acts not subject to prohibition)	Yes*	No	No	Yes	Yes	No	Required	Telecommunications, predetermined plan for emergency
Rhode Island	Traditional	No	—	—	—	—	No	No	No specific legislation	
South Carolina	Traditional	Yes (Applies to "medical" acts only)	Yes	—	—	—	No	Yes	Required	Near proximity, available for consultation

State										
South Dakota	New & Additional Acts Amendment	No	Yes	Yes	Yes	Yes	No	Yes	Not stated	
Tennessee	Traditional	Yes (Applies to "medical" acts only)	Yes (Plus separate exemption for nurses under physician supervision)	No	—	—	—	—	Required	As indicated in written protocols for specific situations
Texas	Traditional	Yes (Applies to "medical" acts only)	Yes	Yes	—	—	—	Yes	Required (for medical treatment)	
Utah	New & Additional Acts Amendment	No	Yes	No	Yes	—	—	—	Required	
Vermont	New & Additional Acts Amendment	Yes	Yes (Under physician supervision)	Yes	Yes	Yes	Yes	No	No regulations	
Virginia	Traditional (Additional Amendments to Medical Practice Act)	No	Yes (Includes specific reference to certain procedures, which must be performed under orders of physician, plus separate exemption for nurses acting under physician supervision pursuant to rules and regulations of Boards of Nursing and Medicine)	No	—	—	—	Yes	Must be available for consultation	
Washington	New & Additional Acts Amendment	No	No	No	Yes	Yes	Yes*	Yes**	Uses "scope of practice" as in statements by national associations	

If Additional Acts Amendment, Criteria and Conditions Stated

State	Type of Definition	Definition Includes Prohibition Against Acts of Diagnosis and Prescription	Rules and Regulations	Professional Opinion	Education and Training	If New Definition, Incorporated some or all of New York's	Prohibitions of Practice of Medicine in Nurse Practice Act	Exception for Nursing in Medical Practice Act	Physician Supervision of Nurse Practitioners	Degree of Supervision
West Virginia	Traditional	No	—	—	—	—	No	Yes	Required	Nurse anesthetists in presence of physician, nurse-midwives according to ACNM standards
Wisconsin	Traditional	No	—	—	—	—	No	Yes (Under physician supervision)[4]	No specific legislation	
Wyoming	New	No	—	—	—	—	No	Yes (Under physician supervision)	Required	Telecommunications, referral and consultation, regular chart review, pre-determined plan for emergencies, protocols for medication

[1] Arizona's additional acts amendment, unlike any other, describes substantively one such act: the dispensing of prepackaged, labelled drugs under certain limited, specific circumstances.

[2] Hawaii has a delegation provision which applies to "any physician-support personnel" and which could be construed as including nurses.

[3] Although Maryland's additional acts amendment does not mention physician supervision, the amendment could be interpreted as subordinate to the definition's general description of nursing as consisting of "independent" nursing functions and "delegated" medical functions, in which case any medical acts within the additional acts amendment would have to be delegated acts.

[4] North Carolina's additional acts amendment does not mention physician supervision, but it appears in a separate section from the definition and would appear to be subordinate to that provision of the definition which prohibits acts of medical diagnosis and prescription except under physician supervision.

[5] Oregon alone among the states with additional acts amendments which refer to professional opinion speaks only of nursing opinion, as opposed to medical and nursing opinion.

[6] Wisconsin's law in this regard is somewhat oblique, but it would appear that not only nurses but any persons are authorized to "assist" physicians.

*By Boards of Nursing and Medicine.
**By Board of Nursing.
***By Board of Nursing or "in collaboration with" Board of Medicine.

Index